# Periodontal Regeneration

## Current Status and Directions

Edited by

## Alan M. Polson, DDS, MS

Director of Clinical Research
Atrix Laboratories
Fort Collins, Colorado

Clinical Professor of Periodontics
School of Dentistry
University of Colorado
Denver, Colorado

quintessence
books

Quintessence Publishing Co, Inc
Chicago, Berlin, London, Tokyo, Moscow, Prague, Sofia, Warsaw

**Library of Congress Cataloging-in-Publication Data**

Periodontal regeneration : current status and directions /
   [edited by] Alan M. Polson.
       p.   cm.
   Includes bibliographical references and index.
   ISBN 0-86715-175-7
   1. Periodontium—Regeneration.  I. Polson, Alan M.
   [DNLM:  1. Periodontium—physiology.  2. Guided Tissue
Regeneration.  3. Regeneration.  4. Periodontal Disease—surgery.
WU 240 P4466 1994]
RK361.P457   1994
617.6'32—dc20
DNLM/DLC
for Library of Congress                                  93-39373
                                                      CIP

quintessence
books

Composition: Midwest Technical Publications, St. Louis, MO
Printing and binding: Everbest Printing Co, Ltd, Hong Kong
Printed in Hong Kong

# Contents

**This book is dedicated to:**

Anne,
   for her continuous encouragement, understanding, and support. . .

my family,
   for their patience and interest. . .

Helmut Zander,
   for his unique mentorship. . .

and my colleagues,
   for their stimulation and collaboration.

# Contributors

**William Becker, DDS, MSD**
Assistant Professor
Department of Periodontology
School of Dentistry
University of Southern California
Los Angeles, California
*and*
Clinical Professor
Department of Periodontics
Dental Branch
University of Texas
Houston, Texas

**Raul G. Caffesse, DDS, MS, Dr Odont**
Professor and Chairman
Department of Periodontology
University of Texas
Houston, Texas

**Jack G. Caton, DDS, MS**
Professor of Periodontology
Director of Advanced Training Program
    in Periodontics
Department of Periodontology
Eastman Dental Center
Rochester, New York

**Carlo Clauser, MD, DDS**
Private Practice
Florence, Italy

**Pierpaolo Cortellini, MD, DDS**
Assistant Professor
Department of Periodontology
University of Siena
Siena, Italy

**Steven Garrett, DDS, MS**
Private Practice
Redlands, California

**Gary Greenstein, DDS, MS**
Chief of Periodontics
Monmouth Medical Center
Long Branch, New Jersey

**Philip J. Hanes, DDS, MS**
Associate Professor
Department of Periodontics
Medical College of Georgia
Augusta, Georgia

**Samuel E. Lynch, DMD, DMSc**
Executive Director
Research and Development
Institute of Molecular Biology, Inc
Worcester, Massachusetts
*and*
Department of Periodontology
Harvard University
Boston, Massachusetts

**James T. Mellonig, DDS, MS**
Associate Professor
Director, Periodontal Postdoctoral Program
Department of Periodontics
University of Texas
San Antonio, Texas

**Preston D. Miller, Jr, DDS**
Clinical Professor
Department of Periodontics
University of Tennessee
Memphis, Tennessee

7

**Carlos Nasjleti, DDS**
Senior Research Associate
Department of Periodontology
University of Texas
Houston, Texas

**Fusanori Nishimura, MD, PhD**
Associate Research Scientist
Laboratory of Tumor Biology
  and Connective Tissue Research
Bronx Veterans Administration Medical Center
*and*
Department of Pathology
College of Physicians and Surgeons
Columbia University
New York, New York

**Giovanpaolo Pini Prato, MD, DDS**
Professor and Chairman
Department of Periodontology
University of Siena
Siena, Italy

**Alan M. Polson, DDS, MS**
Director of Clinical Research
Atrix Laboratories, Inc
Fort Collins, Colorado
*and*
Clinical Professor of Periodontics
Department of Periodontology
University of Colorado
Denver, Colorado

**Ray M. Price, PhD**
Associate Researc h Scientist
Laboratory of Tumor Biology
  and Connective Tissue Research
Bronx Veterans Administration Medical Center
*and*
Department of Pathology
College of Physicians and Surgeons
Columbia University
New York, New York

**Victor Terranova, DMD, PhD**
Director
Laboratory of Tumor Biology
  and Connective Tissue Research
Bronx Veterans Administration Medical Center
*and*
Associate Professor
Department of Pathology
College of Physicians and Surgeons
Columbia University
New York, New York

**Jiuming Ye, MD, PhD**
Associate Research Scientist
Laboratory of Tumor Biology
  and Connective Tissue Research
Bronx Veterans Administration Medical Center
*and*
Department of Pathology
College of Physicians and Surgeons
Columbia University
New York, New York

**Raymond A. Yukna, DMD, MS**
Professor and Head
Department of Periodontics
Louisiana State University
New Orleans, Louisiana

# Introduction

Alan M. Polson

> If alveoli have really been de-
> stroyed in those cases of loose
> teeth . . . whether they have a
> power of renewing themselves
> analogous to that power by which
> they first grow . . .
>
> —John Hunter (1803)

The challenge of periodontal regeneration has come to the forefront of periodontal research and practice. In the overall evolution of periodontal therapy, initial attention focused upon the arrest of disease and long-term maintenance of the dentition. A convincing number of short- and long-term studies have shown that these goals are attainable, provided that one adheres to certain fundamental principles. Moreover, these results can be achieved by a number of different therapeutic approaches.

Research regarding periodontal therapy has made it clear that standard treatment techniques do not result in periodontal regeneration. It has also become apparent that, if the goal of periodontal regeneration is to be realized, the problem of regeneration needs to be approached from a basic biological perspective.

The periodontium consists of a cell-and-tissue complex organized spatially into the basic components of cementum, periodontal ligament, and alveolar bone. The challenge of regeneration is to reconstitute this complex onto a root surface that is the site of marginal periodontitis.

A great deal of biologically based information relating to periodontal regeneration has been obtained during the last decade. The information has been produced by a number of outstanding researchers and clinicians. Each of these individuals has tended to focus upon a particular tissue component and aspect of the challenge of periodontal regeneration. The advantage of this approach has been that high quality and essential information regarding the role of each particular component has been obtained.

Nevertheless, if the clinical result is to be a successful periodontal regeneration, it can only be achieved by proper understanding and simultaneous management of all tissue and clinical components. This book has been prepared in the hope that it will, in some meaningful way, contribute to the attainment of such an ultimate clinical goal.

In this book, premier investigators and clinicians in different areas wrote a summary of their own particular works and findings. Each addressed biological and clinical considerations and speculated upon periodontal regeneration potentials. Each responded in a magnificent manner, and I wish to express my gratitude to each of them.

The text has been assembled in an order corresponding with evolutionary developments in periodontal regeneration.

After focusing on outcomes of current conventional clinical therapeutic procedures, the role of the root surface and early wound healing events are considered together with clinical approaches that utilize such methods for regeneration. The current status of osseous and synthetic bone grafts are also reviewed.

An alternative approach to regeneration has been to obtain selective cell repopulation in sites by cells that have the progenitor potential to form the necessary structural components of the periodontium (the principle of guided tissue regeneration). Extensive clinical experiences with these techniques are reported together with approaches taken when augmentation factors are used in combination with guided tissue regeneration. In addition, possibilities for the use of resorbable barriers for periodontal regeneration are considered.

One of the more recent approaches to regeneration is to try to control the cellular and molecular bases of regeneration (notably via growth factors). The most current information is presented, together with clinical outcome experiences after using biological mediators in periodontal wound healing situations.

After one has reviewed the depth and scope of the information presented in this book, the complexity of predictable and substantial periodontal regeneration becomes apparent. However, while we improve our knowledge about individual components, future success at the clinical level will depend on an ability to understand and manage the interaction and cascade between the different components. It is hoped that the aggregated information in the following chapters will help facilitate such an interactive process and contribute to the linkage between scientific evidence and success in clinical therapeutic procedures.

> The only rational form of treatment is that which calls forth the recuperative powers of the body . . . .
> —John Hunter (1793)

Chapter 1

# Results of Conventional Therapeutic Techniques for Regeneration

Jack G. Caton / Gary Greenstein

## Introduction

*Periodontitis* is defined as inflammation involving and destroying the supporting alveolar bone and periodontal ligament (American Academy of Periodontology 1986). The cause of periodontitis is bacterial plaque. The *lesion of periodontitis* is characterized by severe inflammation, subgingival plaque and calculus, loss of alveolar bone and periodontal ligament, and apical positioning of the pocket and junctional epithelium (Fig 1-1). Clinically, the lesion is recognized by gingival redness, bleeding, and enlargement or recession. Periodontal pockets that extend apical to the cementoenamel junction are present, and loss of alveolar bone can be viewed in dental radiographs (Caton 1989).

Periodontal therapy for treatment of periodontitis involves the elimination of bacterial plaque. When periodontitis is resolved, an *anatomic defect* remains in the periodontium. This anatomic defect is characterized by reformation of gingival fibers, substantial reduction of inflammation, persistent loss of bone and ligament, and formation of a long

junctional epithelium (Caton and Zander 1976; Caton et al 1980, 1989; Listgarten 1967; Listgarten and Rosenberg 1979; Tagge et al 1975) (Fig 1-2). Clinically, on elimination of subgingival bacterial plaque, substantial changes can be observed. Clinical signs of gingival inflammation, ie, redness and bleeding, disappear. Periodontal pockets are reduced in depth as a result of gingival recession and gain of clinical attachment (Caton et al 1982, 1989; Cercek et al 1983; Proye et al 1982; Tagge et al 1975). However, increased probing depths, loss of clinical attachment, and radiographically observed bone loss remain (Caton 1989). Substantial efforts have been made to alter this anatomic defect as part of periodontal therapy.

Thus, periodontal therapy involves two primary components: elimination of bacterial plaque and elimination of the anatomic defects produced by periodontitis. There are two primary approaches to eliminating these anatomic defects: *resective* and *regenerative*, both surgical. Resective surgery seeks to eliminate periodontal defects by removal of the gingival and bony

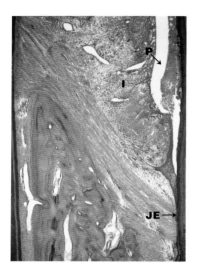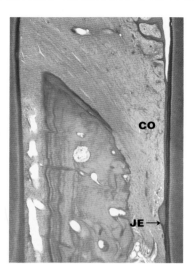

Fig 1-1 *(Left)* The lesion of periodontitis is characterized by subgingival deposits of plaque and calculus *(P)*, severe inflammation *(I)* in the connective tissues and epithelium of the pocket wall, and loss of alveolar bone and periodontal ligament. This allows apical migration of the junctional epithelium *(JE)*. Mesiodistal section of interproximal site, mandibular first molar–second premolar region. (Hematoxylin and eosin stain.)

Fig 1-2 *(Right)* The defect produced by periodontitis remains after resolution of the disease. The inflammatory lesion disappears and is replaced by dense collagenous tissue *(CO)* when subgingival etiologic factors are eliminated. Partial fill of bony defects can occur; however, the junctional epithelium *(JE)* remains in an apical location. This is an example of periodontal repair. Mesiodistal section of interproximal site, mandibular first molar–second premolar region. (Hematoxylin and eosin stain.)

walls; this is accomplished by gingivectomy, osseous resection, and apically positioned flaps (Ochsenbein 1960; Ramfjord et al 1987). Regenerative surgery seeks to eliminate periodontal defects by creating new bone and periodontal ligament and coronally displacing the gingival attachment and margin. This chapter is primarily concerned with periodontal regenerative surgery.

## Regeneration and repair

Periodontal regeneration means healing after periodontal surgery that results in the formation of a new attachment apparatus, consisting of cementum, periodontal ligament, and alveolar bone (Fig 1-3). Periodontal repair implies healing after periodontal surgery without restoration of the normal attachment apparatus. Repair of a periodontal defect can be mediated by formation of a long junctional epithelium and bone fill (Figs 1-4 and 1-5), as well as root resorption (Figs 1-6a and b), ankylosis (Fig 1-7), and fibrous adhesion (Fig 1-8). A combination of these various healing responses often occurs. Thus, increased bone volume and density (bone fill) is commonly observed in angular bony de-

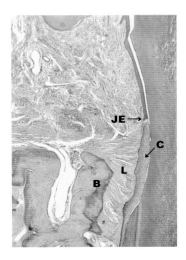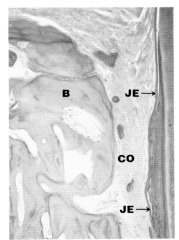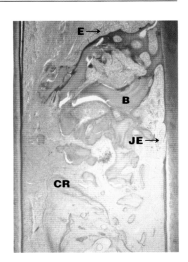

Fig 1-3 *(Left)* Periodontal regeneration has occurred in the apical part of this defect, 1 year after flap surgery. It is characterized by new cementum *(C)* deposited on root-planed dentin and old cementum. New bone *(B)* is connected to the cementum by a new periodontal ligament *(L)*. Apical end junctional epithelium *(JE)*. Mesiodistal section of interproximal site, mandibular first molar–second premolar region. (Hematoxylin and eosin stain.)

Fig 1-4 *(Middle)* Histologic condition 1 year following a modified Widman flap procedure. The inflammatory lesion is absent, new bone *(B)* has completely filled the angular bony defect, and the space between the bone and the root is occupied by dense collageneous tissue *(CO)* that resembles a new periodontal ligament. A long junctional epithelium *(JE)*, however, separates the new bone and connective tissue from the root surface. Mesiodistal section of interproximal site, mandibular first molar–second premolar region. (Hematoxylin and eosin stain.)

Fig 1-5 *(Right)* Histologic condition 1 year following an autogenous bone graft. Transplanted bone *(B)* is present in the area coronal to the alveolar crest *(CR)*. The coronal end of the graft material is partly surrounded by epithelium *(E)*. The apical level of the junctional epithelium *(JE)* is close to the apical level of root planing. Junctional epithelium separates the bone graft from the root surface. Mesiodistal section of interproximal site, mandibular first molar–second premolar region. (Hematoxylin and eosin stain.)

fects in dental radiographs (Polson and Heijl 1978; Rosling et al 1976). Histologic studies have demonstrated, however, that this new bone is usually not connected to the root surface because of an intervening long junctional epithelium (Caton et al 1980; Caton and Zander 1975; Caton and Kowalski 1976) (Fig 1-4). A partial regeneration, that is, a cementum-mediated new fibrous attachment to a pathologically exposed root surface, can also take place without new bone formation.

# Response of the periodontium to therapy

Several types of periodontal treatment have been used to achieve periodontal regeneration. These have traditionally included scaling, root planing, gingival curettage, and various types of flap procedures. Changes reportedly produced by these therapies include pocket depth reduction mediated by gingival recession and gain of clinical attachment. When angular bony defects are

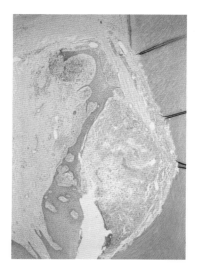
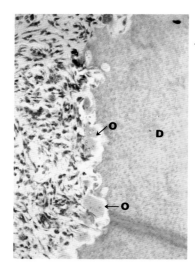

Fig 1-6a   *(Left)* Histologic condition 3 months following transplantation of autogenous red marrow and cancellous bone. An area of active root resorption impedes the apical migration of the epithelium.

Fig 1-6b   *(Right)* Higher magnification of the area of root resorption depicted in Fig 1-6a. Active root resorption is confirmed by the presence of osteoclasts *(O)* in apposition to the dentinal *(D)* surface. Mesiodistal section, maxillary central incisor–lateral incisor region. (Hematoxylin and eosin stain.)

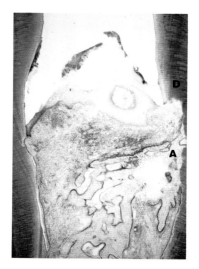
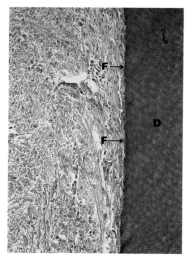

Fig 1-7   *(Left)* Ankylosis *(A)* has occurred, which joins the alveolar bone to the dentin *(D)*, 1 month after transplantation of autogenous red marrow and cancellous bone. Mesiodistal section of interproximal site, mandibular first molar–second premolar region. (Hematoxylin and eosin stain.)

Fig 1-8   *(Right)* A zone of fibrous attachment *(F)* to the dentin root surface *(D)*, not mediated by new cementum formation, was obtained 2 months after acute wounding. Buccolingual section, palatal surface of maxillary second premolar. (Hematoxylin and eosin stain.)

not corrected, they often are remodeled by a process of bone fill and crestal resorption (leveling) (Polson and Heijl 1978).

Until the mid-1970s, the gain of clinical attachment and bone fill produced by conventional periodontal therapy was interpreted to indicate that a true regeneration of the periodontium had occurred. Various substances were placed around teeth and within bony defects prior to flap closure to enhance the bone augmentation. Several longitudinal human clinical trials from research centers around the world have demonstrated that conventional periodontal therapy, followed by good periodontal supportive therapy, is effective in stabilizing periodontal status and maintaining periodontal health (Becker et al 1984; Knowles et al 1979; Lindhe and Nyman 1984; Lindhe et al 1982; Philstrom et al 1983; Ramfjord et al 1987).

The clinical methods of evaluating periodontal therapy are periodontal probing, examination of radiographs, and reentry procedures (Caton 1989). Pretreatment and posttreatment measurements are compared to determine the effect of the therapy. These clinical methods of evaluation, however, cannot distinguish between periodontal repair and periodontal regeneration. A periodontal probe is used to measure pocket (probing) depth, clinical attachment level, and gingival margin location. The *pocket* or *probing depth* is the distance between the gingival margin and the depth of probe tip penetration into the pocket (Caton 1989). The *clinical attachment level* is the distance between the cementoenamel junction and the apical depth of probe tip penetration into the pocket (Caton 1989). *Gingival margin location* is the distance between the gingival margin and the cementoenamel junction (gingival margin location measures the degree of recession).

Clinical attachment level measurements are important in evaluation of therapies

designed to regenerate a new periodontium to the root surface that has been exposed to a periodontal pocket. While this is the best clinical measure, current opinion is that probing cannot accurately measure the connective tissue attachment level, ie, the coronal level of the periodontal ligament. Large gains in clinical attachment can occur after therapy without regeneration of new periodontal ligament. These "false" gains are the result of resolution of inflammation, bone fill, reformation of the gingival collagen fibers, and formation of a long junctional epithelium (Caton et al 1980) (Fig 1-2). Therefore, probing methods are not adequate to evaluate periodontal regenerative therapies (Greenstein 1984; Listgarten 1980).

Reentry procedures typically involve reflecting a flap sometime after initial therapy to compare new bone levels to initial bone levels. While the gross behavior of bone can be measured by this method, bone measurements do not reflect connective tissue attachment levels and cannot distinguish bone that is attached to the root surface via a periodontal ligament and are, therefore, inappropriate for evaluation of periodontal regenerative therapy (Caton and Zander 1976). Similarly, changes in bone height, density, and volume can be estimated by comparison of pretreatment and posttreatment radiographs, but radiographs cannot reveal if the bone is connected to the tooth by new periodontal ligament and cementum (true regeneration) (Caton 1989; Friedman 1958).

Histologic evaluation is the only reliable method to determine the true efficacy of periodontal therapies aimed at creation of a new attachment apparatus consisting of new cementum, bone, and periodontal ligament. Animal models are used for these evaluations because of ethical reasons, the need to limit variation, and the need to provide controls. Many animal models have been utilized with success, but a nonhuman primate model is generally accepted to be the most useful for direct extrapolation of data to humans. Such a model was created by preparing contralateral defects with the same amount of bone and periodontal ligament loss (Caton and Zander 1975; Caton and Kowalski 1976). Typically, the therapy to be tested is done on one side of the arch and results are compared histologically to those on the contralateral side to determine the effect of experimental treatment on levels of bone, cementum, and periodontal ligament. In this way, it can be ascertained whether the experimental treatment produced repair or regeneration. These determinations are especially important for testing the safety and efficacy of new techniques, drugs, and devices (Caton et al 1992).

Results from these controlled animal studies and from evaluation of human block sections have suggested that conventional periodontal surgery results in repair, rather than regeneration (Caton et al 1980; Listgarten and Rosenberg 1979). This knowledge, along with the increasing sophistication of investigators and technologies, led many research laboratories to a systematic and scientific approach to the study of periodontal wound healing. This involved the definition of the variables involved in periodontal wound healing and the experimental manipulation of these variables to solve the riddle of how to achieve periodontal regeneration (Caffesse et al 1985; Gantes et al 1988; Garrett et al 1978; Martin et al 1988; Melcher 1976; Melcher et al 1987; Nyman et al 1982; Polson and Caton 1982; Polson and Proye 1982; Polson 1986; Terranova et al 1986; Terranova and Wikesjö 1987; Wikesjö and Nilvéus 1990). Wound healing variables that have received the most attention include (1) manipulation of progenitor cell populations; (2) alteration of pathologically exposed root surfaces; (3) exclusion of gingival epithelium from the wound; (4) wound stabilization; and (5) technical aspects of dealing with the reduced periodontium, including grafting techniques. A review of the contemporary regenerative therapies that are based on manipulation of these variables follows.

# Progenitor cell populations

For regeneration to occur, cells with the capability to synthesize cementum, bone, and periodontal ligament must occupy the periodontal defect and produce these specialized tissues. It is currently thought that these periodontal progenitor cells reside in the periodontal ligament and/or the alveolar bone remaining around the tooth (Melcher 1976; Melcher et al 1987; Nyman et al 1982).

Devices, bioactive substances, and technical manipulations have been developed to favor repopulation of the periodontal defect by periodontal progenitor cells and discourage repopulation by cells that do not have the capability to produce periodontal supporting tissues. Coronally positioned or anchored flaps delay apical proliferation of gingival epithelium and connective tissue and allow time for coronal migration of periodontal ligament and bone cells (Gantes et al 1988; Garrett et al 1978; Martin et al 1988). Physical barriers made of polytetrafluoroethylene and bioabsorbable materials promote guided tissue regeneration by physically inhibiting gingival epithelium and connective tissue and favoring repopulation of the periodontal defect by cells from the periodontal ligament and alveolar bone (Caton et al 1992) (Figs 1-9a and b). The abilities of growth factors and attachment proteins applied to the periodontal defect to stimulate periodontal progenitor cells and inhibit undesirable cells are being investigated (Terranova et al 1986; Terranova and Wikesjö 1987). Finally, bone augmentation grafts may act as space-maintaining

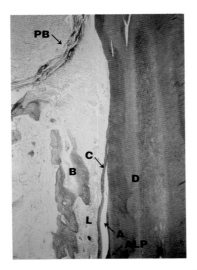 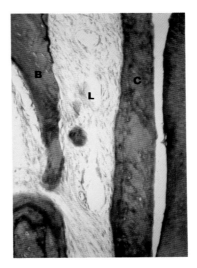

Fig 1-9a    *(Left)* Overview of guided tissue regeneration. New bone *(B)*, cementum *(C)*, and periodontal ligament *(L)* have formed adjacent to root-planed dentin *(D)* surface. Artifactual separation of new cementum from dentin *(A)*; apical level of root planing *(ALP)*; polytetrafluoroethylene barrier *(PB)*.

Fig 1-9b    *(Right)* Higher magnification of an area in Fig 1-9a, showing regeneration of bone *(B)*, periodontal ligament *(L)*, and cementum *(C)*. Mesiodistal section, interproximal area of mesial mandibular first molar. (Hematoxylin and eosin stain.)

devices to allow coronal migration of periodontal progenitor cells.

## Root surface alterations

Periodontitis produces substantial changes of the tooth root surface, and the root is commonly referred to as "pathologically exposed." The normal root is rich in collagen, with extrinsic and intrinsic fibers that form a renewable connection to the adjacent alveolar bone. Plaque-induced inflammation destroys these Sharpey's fibers, allowing downgrowth of junctional and pocket epithelium. Thus, the root surface becomes exposed to the periodontal pocket and oral environment. With loss of collagen, the root surface becomes hypermineralized. Bacterial plaque and calculus

penetrate the cementum and/or dentin of the root (Polson and Caton 1982; Polson 1986). Decalcification and caries can also occur. The root surface thus becomes toxic and unsuitable for the new connective tissue attachment necessary for periodontal regeneration (Polson and Caton 1982).

A critical step in periodontal regenerative therapy is to alter the periodontitis-affected root surface to make it a hospitable substrate to support and encourage migration, attachment, proliferation, and proper phenotypic expression of periodontal connective tissue progenitor cells. Mechanical and chemical means have been used to promote favorable root surface characteristics. These techniques and treatments are discussed in detail elsewhere in this book. Scaling and root planing are used to remove hard and soft deposits and the surface of the cementum and dentin that has been penetrated by these deposits (Cercek et al 1983; Proye et al 1982; Tagge et al 1975). Acids are used to remove the smear layer left by mechanical instrumentation and to expose the intrinsic collagen of the root dentin (Garrett et al 1978; Polson and Proye 1982). Attachment proteins and growth factors are applied to the root surface to stabilize initial clot attachment and encourage periodontal progenitor cells to repopulate the root surface and adjacent clot (Caffesse et al 1985; Terranova et al 1986; Terranova and Wikesjö 1987).

## Epithelial exclusion

When the gingival flap is replaced against the tooth during a periodontal flap procedure, the most aggressive tissue during the initial phases of wound healing is gingival epithelium (Caton and Zander 1976; Caton et al 1980; Listgarten and Rosenberg 1979). Epithelium proliferates apically on the tooth aspect of the flap and becomes attached to the tooth, forming a long junctional epithelium (see Fig 1-2). This effectively prevents connective tissue from gaining access to the root surface and precludes periodontal regeneration. Many techniques, including coronal flap manipulation, fibrin linkage, placement of physical barriers, root submergence, and use of bioactive inhibitory substances, are available to inhibit gingival epithelium.

## Wound stabilization

There is growing evidence that wound stabilization may be a critical variable in the early stages of periodontal wound healing to achieve periodontal regeneration (Gantes et al 1988; Martin et al 1988). When a periodontal flap is replaced, a blood clot is formed between the flap and the root surface. The fibrin of the clot forms the initial attachment to the root surface, preventing epithelial downgrowth and forming a scaffold for development of a cell and collagen fiber attachment mechanism (Polson and Proye 1982; Polson 1986). This initial fibrin attachment to the root surface is easily disturbed and requires protection until it is replaced by collagen fibrils. Flap management techniques and bone augmentation procedures may contribute to wound stabilization.

## Reduced periodontium

Periodontitis destroys the coronal periodontium. The most obvious clinical signs are bone loss and gingival recession. In addition, the periodontal ligament and alveolar bone become located relatively far away from the pathologically exposed root surface, ie, the area where regeneration must take place. Gingival recession presents a significant technical problem for regenerative therapy, and solutions are described in the chapters on flap management and periodontal plastic surgery. Furthermore, bone augmentation grafts have been successfully used to increase the height of the periodontal attachment apparatus.

## Summary

Periodontal therapy involves the elimination of pathogenic bacteria to resolve the inflammatory lesion and the use of resective or regenerative surgery to alter the defects produced by the inflammatory lesions. Conventional periodontal surgery results in repair rather than regeneration. Controlled histologic investigations in laboratory animal models have been crucial to the testing of wound healing variables, critical to achieve periodontal regeneration, and to establishing the safety and efficacy of new devices and bioactive substances.

Thus, a systematic approach to the study of periodontal wound healing has led to innovative methods to achieve periodontal regeneration.

# References

American Academy of Periodontology. Glossary of periodontic terms. *J Periodontol* 1986;57(suppl).

Becker W, Berg LE, Becker BE. The long term evaluation of periodontal treatment and maintenance in 95 patients. *Int J Periodont Rest Dent* 1984; 4(2):54–71.

Caffesse RG, Holden MJ, Kon S, Nasjleti C. The effect of citric acid and fibronectin application on healing following surgical treatment of naturally occurring periodontal disease in beagle dogs. *J Clin Periodontol* 1985;12:578–590.

Caton JG, Zander HA. Primate model for testing periodontal treatment procedures: I. Histologic investigation of localized periodontal pockets produced by orthodontic elastics. *J Periodontol* 1975;46: 71–77.

Caton JG, Kowalski CJ. Primate model for testing periodontal treatment procedures. II. Production of contralaterally similar lesions. *J Periodontol* 1976; 47:506–510.

Caton JG, Zander HA. Osseous repair of an infrabony pocket without new attachment of connective tissue. *J Clin Periodontol* 1976;3:54–58.

Caton J, Nyman S, Zander H. Histometric evaluation of periodontal surgery. II. Connective tissue attachment levels after four regenerative procedures. *J Clin Periodontol* 1980;7:224–231.

Caton J, Proye M, Polson A. Maintenance of healed periodontal pockets after a single episode of root planing. *J Periodontol* 1982;53:420–424.

Caton JG. Periodontal diagnosis and diagnostic aids. In: Nevins R, Becker W, Kornman K, eds. *Proceedings of the World Workshop in Clinical Periodontics.* Chicago: American Academy of Periodontology, 1989:I–32.

Caton J, Bouwsma O, Polson A, Espeland M. Effects of personal oral hygiene and subgingival scaling on bleeding interdental gingiva. *J Periodontol* 1989;60:84–90.

Caton J, Wagener C, Polson A, Nyman S, Frantz B, Bouwsma O, Blieden T. Guided tissue regeneration in interproximal defects in the monkey. *Int J Periodont Rest Dent* 1992;12:267–278.

Cercek JF, Kiger RD, Garrett S, Egelberg J. Relative effects of plaque control and instrumentation on the clinical parameters of human periodontal disease. *J Clin Periodontol* 1983;10:46–56.

Friedman N. Reattachment and roentgenograms. *J Periodontol* 1958;29:98–111.

Gantes B, Martin M, Garrett S, Egelberg J. Treatment of periodontal furcation defects. II. Bone regeneration in mandibular class II defects. *J Clin Periodontol* 1988;15:232–239.

Garrett JS, Crigger M. Egelberg J. Effects of citric acid on diseased root surfaces. *J Periodont Res* 1978;13:155–163.

Greenstein G. The significance of pocket depth measurements. *Compend Contin Educ Dent* 1984; 5:49–52.

Knowles JW, Burgett FG, Nissle RR, Shick RA, Morrison EC, Ramfjord SP. Results of periodontal treatment related to pocket depth and attachment level. Eight years. *J Periodontol* 1979;50: 225–233.

Lindhe J, Westfeld E, Nyman S, Socransky SS, Heijl L, Bratthall G. Healing following surgical/nonsurgical treatment of periodontal disease. *J Clin Periodontol* 1982;9:115–128.

Lindhe J, Nyman S. Long-term maintenance of patients treated for advanced periodontal disease. *J Clin Periodontol* 1984;11:504–514.

Listgarten MA. Electron microscopic features of the newly formed epithelial attachment after gingival surgery. *J Periodont Res* 1967;2:46–52.

Listgarten MA, Rosenberg MM. Histological study of repair following new attachment procedures in human periodontal lesions. *J Periodontol* 1979; 50:333–344.

Listgarten MA. Periodontal probing: What does it mean? *J Clin Periodontol* 1980;7:165–176.

Martin M, Gantes B, Garrett S, Egelberg J. Treatment of periodontal furcation defects (1) Review of the literature and description of a regenerative surgical technique. *J Clin Periodontol* 1988;15:227–231.

Melcher AH. On the repair potential of periodontal tissues. *J Periodontol* 1976;47:256–260.

Melcher AH, McCulloch CAG, Cheong T, Nemeth E, Shiga A. Cells from bone synthesize cementum-like and bone-like tissue in vitro and may migrate into periodontal ligament in vivo. *J Periodont Res* 1987;22:246–247.

Nyman S, Gottlow J, Karring T, Lindhe J. The regenerative potential of the periodontal ligament. An experimental study in the monkey. *J Clin Periodontol* 1982;9:257–265.

Ochsenbein C. Rationale for periodontal osseous surgery. *Dent Clin North Am* 1960;March:27–32.

Philstrom BL, McHugh RB, Oliphant TH, Ortiz-Campos C. Comparison of surgical and nonsurgical treatment of periodontal disease. A review of current studies and additional results after 6½ years. *J Clin Periodontol* 1983;10:524–541.

Polson AM, Heijl LC. Osseous repair in infrabony periodontal defects. *J Clin Periodontol* 1978;5:13–23.

Polson AM, Caton J. Factors influencing periodontal repair and regeneration. *J Periodontol* 1982;53: 617–625.

Polson AM, Proye MP. Effect of root surface alterations on periodontal healing. II. Citric acid treatment of the denuded root. *J Clin Periodontol* 1982; 9:441–450.

Polson AM. The root surface and regeneration; present therapeutic limitations and future biologic potentials. *J Clin Periodontol* 1986;13:995–999.

Proye M, Caton J, Polson A. Initial healing of periodontal pockets after a single episode of root planing monitored by controlled probing forces. *J Periodontol* 1982;53:296–301.

Ramfjord SP, Caffesse RG, Morrison EC, et al. Four modalities of periodontal treatment compared over 5 years. *J Clin Periodontol* 1987;14:445–452.

Rosling B, Nyman S, Lindhe J, Jern B. The healing potential of the periodontal tissues following different techniques of periodontal surgery in plaque-free dentitions. A 2-year clinical study. *J Clin Periodontol* 1976;3:233–250.

Tagge DC, O'Leary TJ, Kafrawy AH. The clinical and histologic response of periodontal pockets to root planing and oral hygiene. *J Periodontol* 1975;46:527–538.

Terranova VP, Aumailley M, Sultan LH, Martin GR, Kleinman HK. Regulation of cell attachment and cell number by fibronectin and laminin. *J Cell Physiol* 1986;127:473–481.

Terranova VP, Wikesjö UME. Extracellular matrices and polypeptide growth factors as mediators of functions of cells of the periodontium. A review. *J Periodontol* 1987;58:371–380.

Wikesjö UME, Nilvéus R. Periodontal repair in dogs: Effect of wound stabilization on healing. *J Periodontol* 1990;61:719–724.

Chapter 2

# The Root Surface and Periodontal Regeneration

Alan M. Polson / Philip J. Hanes

Periodontal therapy has an ultimate goal of predictable regeneration of a periodontium at the site of previous marginal periodontitis (Stahl 1977). A major factor inhibiting predictable regeneration appears to be the nature of the periodontitis-affected root surface. The exposed root surface associated with periodontitis undergoes substantial alterations—the fiber attachment system is destroyed, resulting in a denuded and contaminated root surface (Eide et al 1983, 1984; Selvig 1969; Shackleford 1971). Controlled histologic studies have shown that conventional periodontal treatment procedures do not result in new connective tissue attachment or periodontal regeneration (Caton and Zander 1976, 1979; Caton and Nyman 1980; Caton et al 1980). Consequently, it is necessary to think in more basic and biologic terms about the problem of periodontal regeneration.

## Biologic considerations relating to periodontal regeneration

Several biologic considerations are involved in obtaining new connective tissue attachment to a periodontally diseased root surface. First, the reduced periodontium (as a result of the disease process) may have a limited potential for forming the structural components of a new periodontium, namely, cementum, periodontal ligament, and alveolar bone. The cell populations that now occupy the area previously occupied by the periodontium may no longer have the progenitor populations capable of forming a periodontium. Another factor affecting regenerative potential is that the exposed root surface has undergone substantial alterations and changes; these changes may inhibit formation of a new attachment to the affected root surface. Finally, if pocket epithelium is removed during surgical therapy and the connective tissue is apposed against the root surface, epithelium tends to migrate between the connective tissue and the exposed root surface, thereby precluding a new connective tissue attachment. Thus, several factors within this environment may have a significant biologic influence on the potential for periodontal regeneration. To clarify one aspect of regeneration, an investigation was undertaken to address the relative impor-

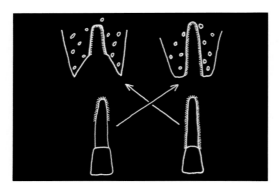

Fig 2-1 Experimental design: The periodontitis-affected maxillary central incisor with the exposed root surface was extracted from the reduced periodontium *(left side)*, and the normal central incisor was extracted from the normal periodontium *(right side)*. The potential for the exposed root surface of the periodontitis-affected tooth to have new connective tissue attachment was evaluated by transplanting that tooth to the normal periodontium. The regenerative capacity of the reduced periodontium was evaluated by transplanting the central incisor with the normal root surface to the reduced periodontium.

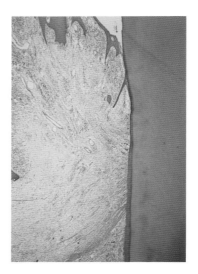

Fig 2-2 Normal root transplanted into reduced periodontium: supracrestal region. Connective tissue reattachment has occurred to the pre-existing level on this normal root surface, although it had been transplanted to a reduced periodontium. (Hematoxylin and eosin stain; original magnification × 10.)

tance of the reduced periodontium and the altered root surface in periodontal healing (Polson and Caton 1982). Experimental periodontitis was produced around a single maxillary central incisor in rhesus monkeys, and both central incisors were extracted and autotransplanted. The regenerative potential of the reduced periodontium was evaluated by transplanting the central incisor with the normal root surface in the reduced periodontium; the potential for obtaining a new connective tissue attachment to the exposed root surface was evaluated by transplanting the diseased root in the normal periodontium (Fig 2-1). The teeth were splinted and evaluated 40 days after transplantation. Radiographic comparisons between the time of transplantation and the end of the evaluation period showed that crestal alveolar bone loss was

associated with the periodontitis-affected root that had been placed into the normal periodontium.

In the group in which the *normal* root had been autotransplanted into the *reduced* periodontium (to evaluate the regenerative potential of the periodontium), the apical end of the sulcular epithelium approximated the level of the cementoenamel junction (CEJ), indicating that connective tissue reattachment had occurred to the preexisting level on this normal root surface even though it had been transplanted into a reduced periodontium (Fig 2-2). The fiber morphology in the supracrestal region showed continuity between the fibers attached to the cementum and those of the adjacent connective tissue. Prior to autotransplantation, the coronal periodontium of the reduced periodontium had an angular

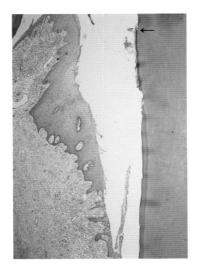 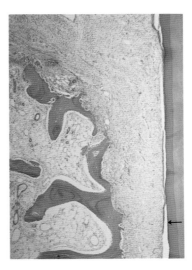

Fig 2-3a and b   Periodontitis-affected root transplanted into normal periodontium.

Fig 2-3a   *(Left)* Epithelium extends along coronal root surface and apical to the cementoenamel junction *(arrow)*. (Original magnification × 10.)

Fig 2-3b   *(Right)* Epithelium lining root surface and terminating *(arrow)* apical to crest of alveolar bone, indicating that a new connective tissue attachment had not occurred on the periodontitis-affected root, although it had been put in a normal periodontium. (Hematoxylin and eosin stain; original magnification × 12.8.)

bony defect morphology. After autotransplantation, remnants of this morphology were still present; however, new bone formation had taken place in the defect and at the alveolar crest. The periodontal ligament had an oriented cell and fiber system, and new cementum was present.

Examination of the *periodontitis-affected roots* that had been autotransplanted into the *normal* periodontium (to evaluate the potential for new connective tissue attachment to the diseased roots) showed that the epithelium that lined the sulcus extended in an apical direction along the cementum surface, and terminated at a point considerably apical to the crest of the alveolar bone (Figs 2-3a and b). This observation indicated that a new connective tissue attachment had not occurred with the periodontitis-affected root even though it had been put in a normal periodontium, one that theoretically had progenitor populations capable of forming the components of a periodontium. Active bone resorption was taking place at the crest of the alveolar bone and corresponded to the radiographic changes observed. Apical to the end of the epithelium on the root surface, the periodontal ligament was reconstituted; presumably this was in an area where attached connective tissue fibers had been present on the root surface at the time of transplantation.

The results of this study clarified the roles of the reduced periodontium and the root surface. Placement of a normal root in a reduced periodontium resulted in a connective tissue reattachment between the fibers on the normal root surface and the adjacent connective tissue fibers—even though the connective tissue fibers were in a supracrestal location and associated with a reduced periodontium. In the periodontitis-affected specimens placed into the normal periodontium, there was no reattachment of fibers to the exposed root surface, and no new connective tissue attachment was generated from the normal periodontium. This indicates that it was the exposed root surface, not lack of a periodontium, that inhibited the potential for a new connective tissue attachment.

# The root surface and periodontal regeneration

Because the altered root surface is a major factor inhibiting regeneration and new attachment, it was decided to evaluate the effect of selective root surface alterations on periodontal healing. The goal was to produce a defined root surface alteration and then study healing in an environment containing periodontal progenitor cells, thereby ensuring that the lack of a progenitor cell population was not affecting the interpretation of the significance of the root surface.

Because the role of attached fibers on the root surface seemed of major importance (Polson and Caton 1982), these studies were initially directed toward evaluating the consequences of fiber denudation and the effect of subsequent surface demineralization of the denuded root surface. In these investigations (Proye and Polson 1982a, 1982b; Polson and Proye 1982), 36 teeth were extracted from squirrel monkeys and divided into three equal groups. In the first group, 12 teeth were reimplanted into their own sockets after the extraction to ascertain the effect of extraction and reimplantation. In the second group, the coronal third of the root surface was planed to remove attached fibers and

cementum (a surgical denudation), and the teeth were replanted into their own sockets. In the third group, the coronal third was root planed, citric acid was applied (pH 1 for 3 minutes), and the teeth were then reimplanted into their own sockets. Total time elapsed with tooth extraction, root instrumentation, acid application, and reimplantation was less than 18 minutes. Specimens were examined 1, 3, 7, and 21 days after reimplantation.

On the clinical level, there were no observable differences in the healing of the gingival tissues around the reimplanted teeth among any of the groups. No form of tooth stabilization had been used, and no teeth exfoliated. Histologic examination of the supracrestal and periodontal ligament regions of the teeth that had only been extracted and reimplanted showed, at 1 day, severe disruption, compared with corresponding regions from normal specimens. These regions in reimplanted specimens exhibited a marked decrease in cellularity and a distinct break in continuity between those fibers remaining attached to the root surface and those attached to the alveolar bone and supracrestal region. The line of fiber cleavage occurred approximately in the middle of the periodontal ligament. Examination of the subsequent healing in this reimplanted group established that, at 21 days, the supracrestal and ligament regions had been reconstituted and there had been *no loss of connective tissue attachment to the root surface.*

The specimens that had been root planed prior to reimplantation demonstrated lack of cementum on the dentin surface, and, at 1 day, the apical end of the sulcular epithelium approximated the original level of the CEJ (Fig 2-4). A cellular fibrin clot occupied the space between the instrumented root surface and the ends of the torn connective tissue fibers. The interface of the fibrin and the root surface

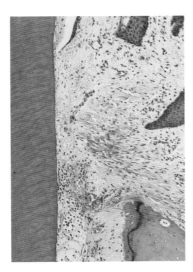

Fig 2-4 Root-planed specimen: supracrestal region, 1 day after reimplantation. (Hematoxylin and eosin stain; original magnification × 40.)

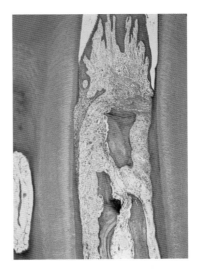

Fig 2-5 Root-planed specimen: supracrestal region and coronal periodontal ligament, 7 days after reimplantation. (Hematoxylin and eosin stain; original magnification × 16.)

was characterized by a lacelike fibrin network that seemed to be apposed against the root surface. Three days after reimplantation, the sulcular epithelium had migrated adjacent to the denuded root surface and its termination was apical to the crest of the alveolar bone. The 7- and 21-day specimens showed epithelial termination apical to the alveolar crest and coinciding with the original apical limit of root instrumentation (Fig 2-5).

In the third group, in which the surface of the denuded root was demineralized prior to reimplantation, the morphologic characteristics at 1 day were similar to those of the denudation-alone group: the level of the sulcular epithelium approximated the original location of the CEJ, the instrumented root surface lacked cementum, and a fibrin clot was interposed between the instrumented surface and the torn ends of the connective tissue fibers (Fig 2-6). Examination of the interface of

the fibrin and the root surface, however, revealed an apparent fibrin attachment to the root surface, mediated by arcadelike fibrin structures. A lighter-staining zone on the surface of the dentin corresponded to the zone of surface demineralization after application of the citric acid. Three days after implantation, the end of the sulcular epithelium still approximated the original level of CEJ; this contrasted markedly with the denudation-alone specimens, in which active apical migration had been apparent. The fibrin clot was still present, attached to the root surface, and seemed to provide a barrier to the migrating epithelium. At all subsequent time points in this group, the epithelium remained at approximately the original level of the CEJ, and a connective tissue fiber attachment system occurred on the instrumented root surface (Fig 2-7).

It was concluded from this series of studies that remnants of connective tissue fibers on the root surface result in a reat-

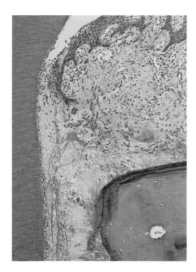

Fig 2-6   Root-planed plus citric acid–treated specimen: supracrestal region and coronal periodontal ligament, 1 day after reimplantation. (Hematoxylin and eosin stain; original magnification × 40.)

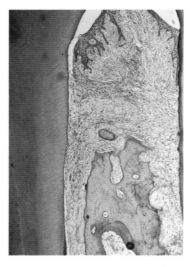

Fig 2-7   Root-planed plus citric acid–treated specimen: coronal periodontium, 7 days after reimplantation. (Hematoxylin and eosin stain; original magnification × 16.)

tachment between the connective tissues, whereas surgical denudation of the root surface (removing attached fibers and cementum) results in epithelial migration and no connective tissue attachment to the root. However, surface demineralization of the denuded root completely changed the wound healing response and resulted in formation of a new connective tissue attachment. It appeared that critical events for this new connective tissue attachment occurred early in the wound healing process. The process seemed to be facilitated by an initial fibrin linkage to the root surface, and these early events occurred prior to formation of collagen fibers.

The existence of a fibrin-collagen cascade that predisposes roots to a new connective tissue attachment had not previously been described. Consequently, a study was undertaken to investigate the chronologic healing sequence of fibrin and

collagen interactions during wound healing (Polson and Proye 1983). Using methodologies similar to those of previous studies, teeth were either root planed and reimplanted, or root planed, acid treated, and reimplanted. The major difference between this study and the previous series was that in the histologic analysis, this study used a staining technique which would simultaneously differentiate between fibrin and collagen. In both groups, a fibrin network was found adjacent to the instrumented root surface at 1 day. However, the acid-treated specimens showed a distinct fibrin attachment to the surface, in contrast to the passive apposition present in the other group (Figs 2-8 and 2-9). In the latter specimens, although the fibrin sequentially became replaced by collagen, epithelium had migrated between the fibrin and the root surface and terminated at the apical limit of root instrumentation (Fig 2-10). In

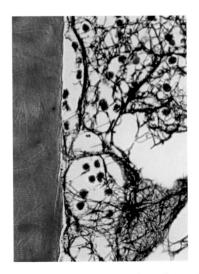 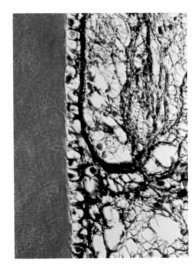

Fig 2-8  *(Left)* Root-planed specimen: interface of the root surface and fibrin, 1 day after reimplantation. The lacelike fibrin network appears to be apposed against the root surface without evidence of physical linkage. (Mallory's phosphotungstic acid–hematoxylin stain; original magnification × 205.)

Fig 2-9  *(Right)* Root-planed plus citric acid–treated specimen: interface of the root surface and fibrin network, 1 day after reimplantation. The fibrin appears to be attached to the root surface by arcadelike structures enclosing inflammatory cells. (Mallory's phosphotungstic acid–hematoxylin stain; original magnification × 205.)

contrast, in the acid-treated specimens, the oriented and attached fibrinous network was replaced by collagen without apical migration of the epithelium along the root surface. The collagen fiber attachment was mediated without cementum formation (Fig 2-11). Thus, it appeared that the fibrin had mediated an initial attachment of the gingival tissues to the root surface and that this matrix of fibrin had served as a scaffolding for cell migration and attachment and subsequent collagen synthesis.

Because demineralization of the denuded root surface had a profound influence on the wound healing process, it was decided to examine the morphology of the denuded root surface before and after surface demineralization by using scanning electron microscopy (Polson et al 1984).

Inspection of the denuded dentin surface prior to demineralization did not reveal orifices of dentinal tubules—an amorphous crustlike material corresponding to a smear layer was present (Fig 2-12). The citric acid–demineralized surface was markedly different in appearance. Numerous funnel-shaped depressions that seemed to correspond to the openings of dentinal tubules were present (Fig 2-13). The overall root surface appeared to have an undulating, rather than flat, morphology. The surface texture was fibrillar and had a matlike structure (Fig 2-14). This appearance corresponded to the exposed collagen matrix of the dentin subsequent to surface demineralization with citric acid. The collagen matrix, in wound healing, seems to provide a hospitable substrate for cellular attach-

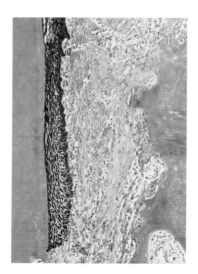 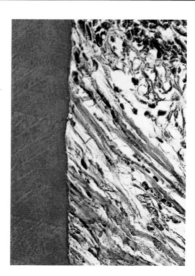

Fig 2-10  *(Left)* Root-planed specimen: coronal periodontal ligament, 21 days after reimplantation. The root-planed surface is lined by epithelium that extends within the ligament space to the limit of root instrumentation. (Mallory's phosphotungstic acid–hematoxylin stain; original magnification × 40.)

Fig 2-11  *(Right)* Root planed plus citric-acid treated specimen 21 days after reimplantation. Collagen fiber attachment to the root surface appears to be present without evidence of cementum formation. (Mallory's phosphotungstic acid–hematoxylin stain; original magnification × 160.)

ment and fiber synthesis and predisposes the wound, therefore, to formation of a new connective tissue attachment.

# The root surface, new attachment, and periodontal progenitor cells

The studies investigating effects of selective root surface alterations on periodontal wound healing indicated that new connective tissue attachment can occur to non–periodontitis-affected root surfaces after removal of cementum and demineralization of the resultant dentin surface. The combination of factors consistent with this new attachment are surface demineralization, close wound adaptation, and an importance of early events during healing.

The regeneration reported in these studies (Polson and Proye 1982, 1983; Proye and Polson 1982a, 1982b) occurred in a tooth-reimplantation model wherein the altered root surfaces had been replanted into a normal periodontium. The normal environment could, conceivably, still have contained periodontal progenitor cells (Melcher 1976). Thus, the role of the root surface in facilitating or inhibiting a connective tissue attachment had to be clarified by studying healing in an environment lacking periodontal progenitor cells. Consequently, an implantation model was developed in which specimens from human root surfaces were implanted into a connective tissue that lacked periodontal progenitor cell populations (Hanes et al 1985).

When a root surface exposed by periodontitis is subjected to conventional me-

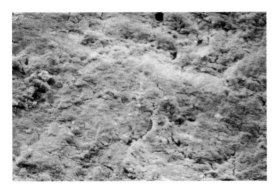

Fig 2-12    Root-planed surface. (Original magnification × 2,110.)

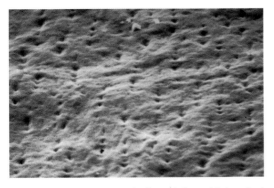

Fig 2-13    Root-planed plus citric acid–treated surface. (Original magnification × 2,110.)

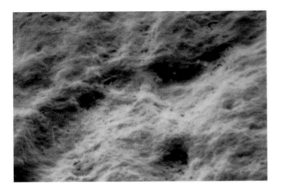

Fig 2-14    Root-planed plus citric acid–treated surface: shallow angle view. (Original magnification × 6,400.)

chanical methods of instrumentation, one of two types of root surface substrates will result: (1) root-planed dentin or (2) scaled and root-planed cementum. Both of these types were originally beneath a periodontitis-affected root surface. Root surface alterations associated with periodontitis have been shown to preclude the development of a new connective tissue attachment, even in the presence of periodontal progenitor cell populations (Polson and Caton 1982). Periodontitis-affected cementum surfaces have loss of collagen fiber insertion (Selvig 1969), show alterations in mineral density (Selvig and Zander 1962; Selvig and Hals 1977), and are contaminated by bacterial endotoxins (Aleo et al 1974, 1975; Hatfield and Baumhammers 1971). Furthermore, it has been shown that microbial (Sottosanti and Garret 1975; Sottosanti 1977; Zander 1953) and endotoxin (Aleo et al 1974, 1975; Bigarre and Yardin 1977; Hatfield and Baumhammers 1971) contamination of exposed cementum may extend to the cementodentinal junction and into the underlying dentin (Adriaens and De Boever 1986; Adriaens et al 1988; Kopczyk and Conroy 1968), suggesting that total mechanical removal of cementum may not totally eliminate etiologic contaminants. In addition, further alterations in the root surface substrate occur following mechanical instrumentation, particularly the development of a surface smear layer (Hanes et al 1986; Jones et al 1972; Polson et al 1984).

To evaluate further the significance of these root surface alterations in periodontal wound healing, an in vivo implantation model was developed in which rectangular specimens obtained from human root surfaces were implanted into incisional wounds in the backs of Sprague-Dawley rats. Root surface specimens of dentin and cementum were obtained from both periodontitis-affected and healthy root surfaces, resulting in four types of root sur-

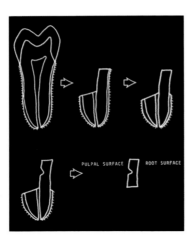

Fig 2-15   Preparation of implant specimens. *(top left)* Extracted, non–periodontitis-affected human tooth with attached periodontal ligament fibers. Specimens for implantation are prepared from areas beneath attached fibers. *(top center)* The crown and root of the tooth coronal to the selected area are resected, and the root is sectioned throughout the pulp canal parallel to the long axis of the tooth. *(top right)* Fibers and cementum are removed from the root surface aspect of the specimen. *(bottom left)* The pulpal surface is notched for clinical and histologic identification. The final specimen is obtained by sectioning at the apical extent of preparation. *(bottom right)* The specimen consists of dentin with distinguishable root and pulpal surface aspects.

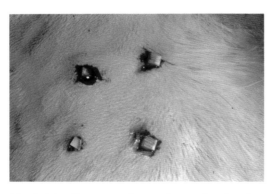

Fig 2-16   Four specimens immediately after they have been implanted into incisional wounds in the skin of a rat. A portion of each implant protrudes above the surface of the skin. The two specimens on the left are non–acid-treated (control), while the two on the right (experimental) were treated with citric acid prior to implantation.

from normal root surfaces (Hanes et al 1985; Hanes and Polson 1989) (Fig 2-15), and from beneath radicular calculus deposits for specimens from periodontitis-affected root surfaces (Polson et al 1986; Polson and Hanes 1989). Half of the specimens were treated with citric acid, pH 1, for 3 minutes, while the remainder served as untreated control specimens. Specimens were implanted transcutaneously through incisional wounds in the skin on the dorsal surface of rats and into the dermal connective tissue (a connective tissue lacking periodontal progenitor cells), so that one end of the implant protruded through the skin (Fig 2-16). Four specimens in each group were available 1, 3, 5, and 10 days after implantation. Histologic and histometric analyses of the healing responses to each of the four type of root surface substrates included counts of adhering cells, evaluation of connective tissue fiber relationships, and assessment of epithelial migration (Hanes et al 1985).

## Dentin from normal root surfaces

To assure the normal, non–periodontitis-affected status of these root surfaces, spec-

face substrates for evaluation: *(1)* normal dentin, *(2)* periodontitis-affected dentin, *(3)* normal cementum, and *(4)* periodontitis-affected cementum.

Rectangular specimens with opposite faces of root and pulpal surfaces were prepared from beneath root surfaces covered by periodontal ligament for specimens

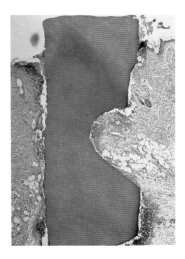 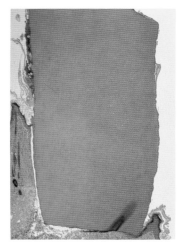 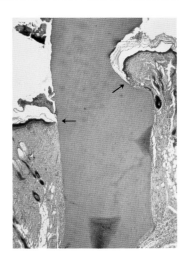

Fig 2-17    *(Left)* Control dentin specimen, 1 day after implantation. Connective tissue is adjacent to the cementum-free root surface and notched pulpal surface aspects of the specimen. One end of the specimen protrudes through the surface of the skin. (Hematoxylin and eosin stain; original magnification × 16.)

Fig 2-18    *(Middle)* Control specimen, 10 days after implantation. (Hematoxylin and eosin stain; original magnification × 12.)

Fig 2-19    *(Right)* Surface-demineralized experimental specimen, 10 days after implantation. The apical termination of the epithelium *(arrows)* corresponds with that present at the time of implantation. (Hematoxylin and eosin stain; original magnification × 10.)

imens were taken from the midroot region, well apical to the coronal extent of attached periodontal ligament fibers (Hanes et al 1985). Remnants of periodontal ligament fibers were removed from the root surface with 12 strokes of a Gracey curet. The cementum was removed with a carborundum disc in a low-speed handpiece.

Following implantation into incisional wounds, analyses within each group, comparing root and pulpal surfaces, showed no differences between any of the parameters. Comparisons between experimental and control groups showed that non–acid-treated control specimens extruded and exfoliated (Figs 2-17 and 2-18), in contrast to the surface-demineralized experimental specimens, which remained within the connective tissue (Fig 2-19). The demineralized surfaces had a greater number of cells attached (Figs 2-20a and b); in addition, fiber attachment occurred (Figs 2-21a and b) and epithelial downgrowth was inhibited. Scanning electron microscopic observations of the early interactions (24 hours) between the dentin surfaces and the connective tissue showed rounded cells on the non-demineralized dentin surfaces, indicating minimal attachment of cells (Figs 2-22 and 2-23), but flattened, elongated cells on demineralized surfaces, suggesting cell

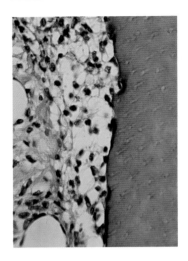 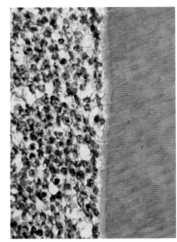

Fig 2-20a *(Left)* Control specimen: interface of root surface and connective tissue, 1 day after implantation. (Hematoxylin and eosin stain; original magnification × 204.)

Fig 2-20b *(Right)* Surface-demineralized experimental specimen: interface of root surface and connective tissue, 1 day after implantation, shows significantly greater cell attachment than does control specimen. (Hematoxylin and eosin stain; original magnification × 204.)

attachment and migration on these acid-treated dentin surfaces (Hanes et al 1988) (Figs 2-24 to 2-26). The fiber attachment to experimental specimens differed morphologically from periodontal ligament fiber attachment to normal root surfaces: the numbers of fibers attached per unit length were fewer and the diameter of attached fibers was smaller on experimental specimens than the corresponding values for normal periodontal ligament fiber attachment. The attachment to these experimental surfaces appeared to have characteristics intrinsic to the connective tissue location.

### Cementum from normal root surfaces

For preparation of cementum specimens from normal roots (Hanes and Polson 1989), remnants of periodontal ligament fibers were removed from the root surface with 12 strokes of a Gracey curet. The remaining cementum on the root surface was not removed.

Following implantation into incisional wounds, epithelial migration was observed adjacent to non–acid-treated cementum surfaces and was associated with extrusion and exfoliation of these control specimens. In contrast, the surface-demineralized experimental specimens remained within the connective tissue (Fig 2-27), and had a cell and fiber attachment system established at 10 days (Figs 2-28a and b). Fiber attachment occurred to both the demineralized cementum and pulpal dentin surfaces, but distinct morphologic differences were apparent in fiber attachment to these two surfaces. Demineralized cementum had fibers that were larger in diameter and had more fibers attached per unit area than did demineralized pulpal dentin surfaces. As was the case with dentin from normal root surfaces, the attachment to demineralized pulpal dentin surfaces appeared to have characteristics intrinsic to the connective tissue location. The larger diameter of the fibers attached to the cementum surfaces suggested that a splicing of Sharpey's fibers within the cementum with fibers in the adjacent connective tissue had been facilitated by exposure of these Sharpey's fibers following acid treatment.

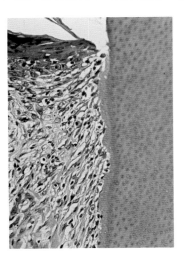

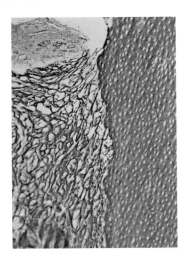

Fig 2-21a  Surface-demineralized experimental specimen: interface of the epithelium, connective tissue, and root surface from Fig 2-19, 10 days after implantation. (Hematoxylin and eosin stain; original magnification × 100.)

Fig 2-21b  Surface-demineralized experimental specimen: interface of the epithelium, connective tissue, and root surface from Fig 2-19, 10 days after implantation, shows connective tissue fiber attachment. (Silver impregnation stain; original magnification × 100.)

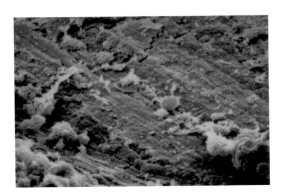

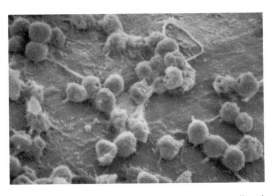

Fig 2-22  Non-demineralized dentinal root surface with large areas devoid of cells or attachments. The surface has an amorphous appearance, and orifices of dentinal tubules are not visible. The globular structures are cells. (Original magnification × 2,100.)

Fig 2-23  Group of cells on non-demineralized surface. The individual cells are rounded, with few processes or extensions. (Original magnification × 6,500.)

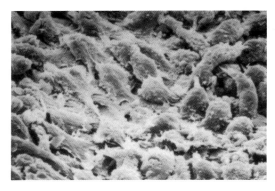

Fig 2-24    Demineralized dentin surface. Numerous cells cover and obscure the underlying dentin surface. (Original magnification × 2,110.)

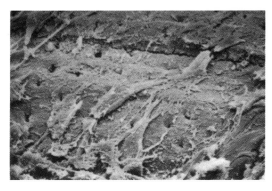

Fig 2-25    Demineralized dentin surface. Attached cells with elongated processes migrate over the dentinal surface substrate. The openings of dentinal tubules are apparent and are distributed throughout the surface area of the dentin. (Original magnification × 1,890.)

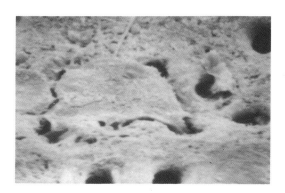

Fig 2-26    Demineralized dentin surface. Cells on the root surface are adjacent to orifices of dentinal tubules and a process extends into a tubule. (Original magnification × 4,200.)

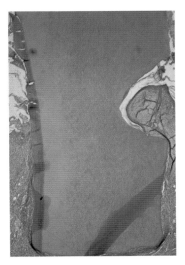
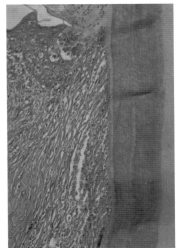
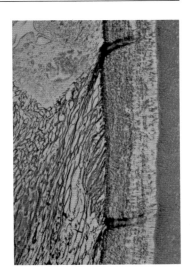

Fig 2-27 Surface-demineralized cementum specimen, 10 days after implantation. (Hematoxylin and eosin stain; original magnification × 16.)

Fig 2-28a *(Left)* Surface demineralized cementum surface: interface of the epithelium, connective tissue, and root surface from Fig 2-27, 10 days after implantation. (Hematoxylin and eosin stain; original magnification × 100.)

Fig 2-28b *(Right)* Surface-demineralized cementum surface: interface of the epithelium, connective tissue, and root surface from Fig 2-27, 10 days after implantation, shows connective tissue fiber attachment. (Silver impregnation stain; original magnification × 100.)

## Dentin from periodontitis-affected root surfaces

To assure the periodontitis-affected nature of these root surfaces, specimens were taken from areas on the root surface beneath deposits of calculus (Polson et al 1986) (Fig 2-29). Calculus was removed from the root surface with an ultrasonic scaler; then the cementum was removed with a carborundum disc in a low-speed handpiece.

Similar to results observed following implantation of specimens of normal dentin, analyses within each group (comparing root and pulpal surfaces) showed no differences between any of the parameters. Comparisons between experimental and control groups showed that non–acid-treated control specimens extruded and exfoliated, in contrast to the surface-demineralized experimental specimens, which remained within the connective tissue (Fig 2-30). The demineralized surfaces had a greater number of cells attached; fiber attachment also occurred and epithelial downgrowth was inhibited (Figs 2-31a and b). The cell and fiber attachment systems associated with the dentin surfaces obtained from periodontitis-affected roots were the same as those associated with dentin surfaces obtained from normal roots (Polson and Hanes 1987). Once again, the connective tissue fiber attachment to demineralized dentin surfaces from periodontitis-affected roots appeared to have characteristics intrinsic to the connective tissue location.

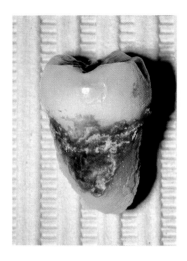 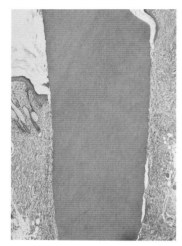

Fig 2-29 *(Left)* Extracted periodontitis-affected tooth with calculus deposits on the root surface. Specimens were taken from areas beneath the calculus deposits.

Fig 2-30 *(Right)* Surface-demineralized dentin from periodontitis-affected root surface, 10 days after implantation. (Hematoxylin and eosin stain; original magnification × 10.)

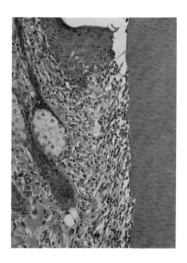 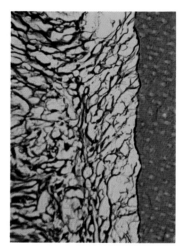

Fig 2-31a and b Area at epithelium, connective tissue, and root surface interface from Fig 2-30.

Fig 2-31a *(Left)* A cell attachment system is present. (Hematoxylin and eosin stain; original magnification × 100.)

Fig 2-31b *(Right)* A fiber attachment system is present. (Silver impregnation stain; original magnification × 100.)

## Cementum from periodontitis-affected root surfaces

Cementum specimens were harvested from areas on the root beneath deposits of calculus (Polson and Hanes 1989). Calculus was removed carefully with an ultrasonic scaler, so that the underlying root surface was not gouged.

Unlike that observed on both root and pulpal surfaces in the previous three studies

(and the pulpal dentin surface in this study), a distinct zone of surface demineralization was not apparent on these periodontitis-affected cementum surfaces following acid treatment (Fig 2-32). In addition, epithelial downgrowth and connective tissue cell and fiber attachment did not differ between experimental and control surfaces at any time in this group (Figs 2-33 and 2-34).

The findings of this study suggested that the periodontitis-affected root surface

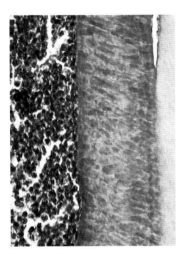 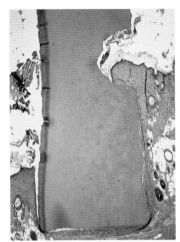 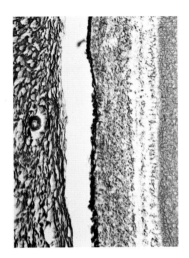

Fig 2-32   *(Left)* Lack of surface demineralization present on cementum surface from periodontitis-affected root surface, 1 day postimplantation. (Hematoxylin and eosin stain; original magnification × 100.)

Fig 2-33   *(Middle)* Surface-demineralized cementum surface implant from beneath periodontitis-affected root surface, 10 days after implantation. Specimen is exfoliating and no cell and fiber attachment system has developed. (Hematoxylin and eosin stain; original magnification × 10.)

Fig 2-34   *(Right)* Cementum surface from Fig 2-33. No fiber attachment. (Silver impregnation stain; original magnification × 100.)

inhibited the demineralization effects of the citric acid.

To evaluate further the differences in cementum surface characteristics after citric acid treatment of cementum from both normal and periodontitis-affected root surfaces, these surfaces were examined with scanning electron microscopes (Hanes et al 1991). Citric acid treatment of cementum from normal root surfaces produced a markedly fibrillar surface morphology that was consistent with the exposure of a fibril-lar, collagen substrate (Fig 2-35). Periodontitis-affected cementum, however, was not appreciably altered in appearance, having only a faintly matlike surface texture (Fig 2-36). These findings suggest that calculus-covered, periodontitis-affected cementum undergoes changes that reduce the effects of the demineralizing agent; this factor may contribute to the inconsistent findings associated with the clinical use of citric acid treatment for the purpose of obtaining new connective tissue attachment.

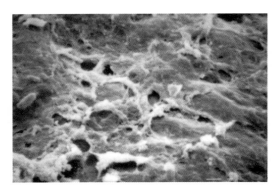
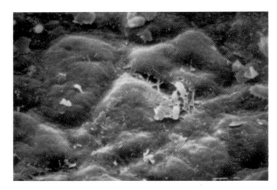

Fig 2-35   *(Left)* Citric acid–treated cementum surface from normal root. The surface morphology is undulating, with a fibrillar, matlike appearance resembling exposed collagen. (Original magnification × 6,400.)

Fig 2-36   *(Right)* Citric acid–treated cementum from periodontitis-affected root. The ovoid mounds are characterized by a faint matlike appearance. Although the magnification is the same as that of Fig 2-35, individual, discrete collagen fibrils are not apparent. (Original magnification × 6,400.)

## Summary

The primary aim of this series of studies was to evaluate early events in healing adjacent to various root surface substrates that were placed in a connective tissue environment that lacked periodontal ligament progenitor cell populations, but included epithelial and connective tissue interactions analogous to those present adjacent to root surfaces after routine periodontal surgical procedures. An implantation model was developed and implemented for this purpose. Early events in healing (1 to 10 days), encompassing epithelial migration and the development of a connective tissue cell and fiber attachment to the root surface(s), were observed. It was concluded that connective tissue cell and fiber attachment can occur to cementum and dentin from normal root surfaces and to dentin from periodontitis-affected root surfaces following citric acid treatment of these surfaces. The morphology of this cell and fiber attachment system differed from that of the normal periodontal ligament attachment, having morphologic characteristics more closely related to the connective tissue associated with this implantation model. The consistent observation of connective tissue fiber attachment to these various root surface substrates in an environment lacking periodontal progenitor cells indicated, however, that this connective tissue can attach to a root surface that has appropriate substrate characteristics.

In contrast to acid-treated dentin surfaces (from both normal and periodontitis-affected roots), and acid-treated cementum from normal roots, periodontitis-affected cementum apparently inhibited the development of a connective tissue cell and fiber attachment system resulting in epithelial migration, extrusion, and exfoliation of the specimens. This lack of connective tissue attachment may be a result of inadequate root preparation. Periodontitis-affected cementum specimens were only scaled with an ultrasonic scaler to remove visible calculus deposits. Etiologic contaminants present in the cementum may have precluded optimal healing responses. Another explanation for this lack of connective tissue attachment may be that the periodontitis-affected cementum inhibited the demineralizing effects of the citric acid. In this regard, previous studies have reported hypermineralization of periodontitis-affected cementum.

Results of the present series of studies support the concept of an inhibition of surface demineralization of periodontitis-affected cementum because significant exposure of collagen matrix was lacking in scanning electron microscopic observations of these surfaces following citric acid treatment. These findings suggest that thorough root planing of the cementum to remove surface contaminants and superficial layers of hypermineralized cementum may be indicated when techniques of root surface conditioning are employed. In this way, potential exposure of a hospitable substrate of cell and fiber attachment would be enhanced.

## Acknowledgments

Investigations from our laboratories reported in this paper were supported by NIDR grant Nos. DE-1648 and DE-7061 and by the Pluta Periodontal Fund.

## References

Adriaens PA, De Boever JA. Ultrastructural study of bacterial invasion in roots of periodontally diseased, caries-free human teeth. J Dent Res 1986;65:770–774.

Adriaens PA, De Boever JA, Loesche WJ. Bacterial invasion in root cementum and radicular dentin of periodontally diseased teeth in humans. A reservoir of periodontopathic bacteria. J Periodontol 1988;59:222–230.

Aleo JJ, De Renzis FA, Farber PA, Varboncoeur AP. The presence and biological activity of cementum-bound endotoxin. J Periodontol 1974;45:672–675.

Aleo JJ, De Renzis FA, Farber PA. In vitro attachment of human gingival fibroblasts to root surfaces. J Periodontol 1975;46:639–645.

Bigarre C, Yardin M. Demonstration of lipids in the pathologic granules in cementum and dentin in periodontal disease. J Clin Periodontol 1977;4:210–213.

Caton JC, Zander HA. Osseous repair of an infrabony pocket without new attachment of connective tissue. J Clin Periodontol 1976;3:54–58.

Caton JG, Zander HA. The attachment between tooth and gingival tissues after periodic root planing and soft tissue curettage. J Periodontol 1979;50:462–466.

Caton J, Nyman S. Histometric evaluation of periodontal surgery. I. The modified Widman flap procedure. J Clin Periodontol 1980;7:212–223.

Caton J, Nyman S, Zander H. Histometric evaluation of periodontal surgery. II. Connective tissue attachment levels after four regenerative procedures. J Clin Periodontol 1980;7:224–231.

Eide B, Lie T, Selvig KA. Surface coatings on dental cementum incident to periodontal disease. I. A scanning electron microscopic study. J Clin Periodontol 1983;10:157–171.

Eide B, Lie T, Selvig KA. Surface coatings on dental cementum incident to periodontal disease. II. Scanning electron microscopic confirmation of a mineralized cuticle. J Clin Periodontol 1984;11:565–575.

Hanes PJ, Polson AM, Ladenheim S. Cell and fiber attachment to demineralized dentin from normal root surfaces. J Periodontol 1985;56:752–765.

Hanes PJ, Polson AM, Frederick GT. Root and pulpal dentin after surface demineralization. Endod Dent Traumatol 1986;2:190–195.

Hanes PJ, Polson AM, Frederick GT. Initial wound healing attachments to demineralized dentin. J Periodontol 1988;59:176–183.

Hanes PJ, Polson AM. Cell and fiber attachment to demineralized cementum from normal root surfaces. J Periodontol 1989;60:188–198.

Hanes PJ, Polson AM, Frederick GT. Citric acid treatment of periodontitis-affected cementum. A scanning electron microscopic study. J Clin Periodontol 1991;18:567–575.

Hatfield CJ, Baumhammers A. Cytotoxic effects of periodontally involved surfaces of human teeth. Arch Oral Biology 1971;16:465–468.

Jones SJ, Lozdan J, Boyde A. Tooth surfaces treated in situ with periodontal instruments. SEM studies. Br Dent J 1972;132:57–63.

Kopczyk R, Conroy C. The attachment of calculus to root planed surfaces. Periodontics 1968;6:78–83.

Melcher AH. On the repair potential of periodontal tissues. J Periodontol 1976;47:256–260.

Polson AM, Caton JC. Factors influencing periodontal repair and regeneration. J Periodontol 1982;53:617–626.

Polson AM, Proye MP. Effect of root surface alterations on periodontal healing. II. Citric acid treatment of the denuded root. J Clin Periodontol 1982;9:441–454.

Polson AM, Proye MP. Fibrin linkage: A precursor for new attachment. J Periodontol 1983;54:141–147.

Polson AM, Frederick GT, Ladenheim S, Hanes PJ. The production of a root surface smear layer by instrumentation and its removal by citric acid. J Periodontol 1984;55:443–446.

Polson AM, Ladenheim S, Hanes PJ. Cell and fiber attachment to demineralized dentin from periodontitis-affected root surfaces. *J Periodontol* 1986;57:235–246.

Polson AM, Hanes PJ. Cell and fiber attachment to demineralized dentin: A comparison between normal and periodontitis-affected root surfaces. *J Clin Periodontol* 1987;14:357–365.

Polson AM, Hanes PJ. Cell and fiber responses to demineralized cementum from periodontitis-affected root surfaces. *J Clin Periodontol* 1989;16:489–497.

Proye MP, Polson AM. Repair in different zones of the periodontium after tooth reimplantation. *J Periodontol* 1982a;53:379–389.

Proye MP, Polson AM. Effect of root surface alterations on periodontal healing. I. Surgical denudation. *J Clin Periodontol* 1982b;9:428–440.

Selvig KA, Zander HA. Chemical analysis and microradiography of cementum and dentin from periodontally diseased human teeth. *J Periodontol* 1962;33:303–310.

Selvig KA. Biological changes at the tooth saliva interface in periodontal disease. *J Dent Res* 1969;48:846–855.

Selvig KA, Hals D. Periodontally diseased cementum studied by correlated microradiography, electron probe analysis and electron microscopy. *J Periodont Res* 1977;12:419–429.

Shackleford JM. Scanning electron microscopy of the dog periodontium. *J Periodont Res* 1971;6:45–54.

Sottosanti J, Garrett J. A rationale for root preparation—a scanning electron microscopic study of diseased cementum. *J Periodontol* 1975;46:628–629.

Sottosanti J. A possible relationship between occlusion, root resorption and the progression of periodontal disease. *J Western Soc Periodontol* 1977;25:69–74.

Stahl SS. Repair potential of the soft tissue-root interface. *J Periodontol* 1977;48:545–552.

Zander HA. The attachment of calculus to root surfaces. *J Periodontol* 1953;24:16–19.

# Chapter 3

# Early Wound Healing Stability and Its Importance in Periodontal Regeneration

Steven Garrett

## Historical perspective

Before periodontal regeneration can be discussed, several terms must be defined. *Regenerative therapy* refers to those procedures that are designed to achieve replacement of lost periodontal tissues. *Regeneration* is the biologic process by which the architecture and function of lost tissues are completely restored. In the case of periodontal treatment, then, regeneration means restitution of lost tooth-supporting tissues, including new alveolar bone, a new periodontal ligament, and gingival structures. *New connective tissue attachment* is the reunion of connective tissue with a root surface that has been pathologically exposed. *Reattachment* is the reunion of connective tissue and a root surface that have been separated by incision or injury. *Bone fill* is defined as the clinical restoration of bone tissue in a previously treated periodontal defect. The term *bone fill* does not address the presence or absence of histologic evidence of new connective tissue attachment or the formation of a new periodontal ligament.

Active periodontitis results in the loss of the tooth's supporting apparatus and eventually in the loss of the tooth. For teeth whose function requires additional periodontal support, or where elimination of periodontal defects will enhance long-term survival, treatment of periodontitis should involve not only the control of further breakdown by eliminating periodontal infection, but also the regeneration of previously lost periodontal support. Current treatment procedures seem insufficient to produce the proper conditions in the healing periodontal surgical wound that lead to complete regeneration. Researchers have found conclusive evidence that a limited amount of regeneration and new connective tissue attachment may occur (Bowers et al 1989; Cole et al 1980) but substantial regeneration is not a predictable outcome of most regenerative attempts, regardless of the therapeutic modality used (Egelberg 1987; Hancock 1989).

Traditionally, treatment of periodontally diseased sites has included surgical exposure of the area, thorough debridement of the diseased site and the adjacent involved root surface, and surgical closure. These procedures generally are effective in controlling the periodontal infection but do not lead to periodontal regeneration. Defects treated in such a manner routinely heal with a long junctional epithelium to the base of the original periodontal pocket (Steiner et al 1981). Even with substantial bone fill in the defect, epithelium may be found between the bone and the root surface (Listgarten and Rosenberg 1979). From these experiences has developed an experimental hypothesis that apical migration of the gingival epithelium must be prevented in order for new connective tissue attachment to the root surface to be achieved. Current regenerative techniques may include efforts to impede apical migration of the epithelium as well as to provide an environment more favorable to regeneration than that provided by conventional periodontal surgery.

All healing wounds proceed through a number of well-defined steps during the process of repair following injury. These have been categorized into three phases: (1) inflammation, (2) fibroblastic-granulation, and (3) matrix formation and remodeling (Clark 1988). The sequencing of these events may be very important in periodontal regeneration. For example, during the early phase of repair, a fibrin clot is formed. In epidermal wounds, this fibrin clot bridges the space between two vascular wound margins and serves as a base that epithelial cells migrate across to cover the wound, providing protection to the underlying connective tissue as healing progresses (Clark 1988). In epidermal wounds, this epithelial proliferation begins approximately 24 hours after injury.

Periodontal surgical wounds during regenerative attempts follow a similar healing pattern, but there are differences in this specific wound healing environment that may affect the outcome of the procedures. When periodontal wounds are closed and

sutured, one of the wound margins is an avascular and rigid root surface. In addition, the healing site, because of the tooth, communicates with the oral environment during all phases of wound healing. Wound healing in this environment generally produces a different result than is found in epidermal sites. Here the epithelium routinely migrates along the inner surface of the wound; the end result is a long junctional epithelium interface with the root surface.

## Research results: early wound healing events

A review of research involving early wound healing events in periodontal wounds indicates that this long junctional epithelium healing pattern should not be the anticipated result. Polson and Proye (1983) used an extraction and reimplantation model in monkeys to study early wound healing. Teeth were extracted; the coronal third of the root was carefully planed; and half of the root-planed teeth were demineralized with citric acid and then reimplanted in their extraction sites. Observations of healing were made at 1, 3, 7, and 21 days. At 1 day all specimens had a fibrin clot adhering to the root surface. However, by 3 days in the nondemineralized specimens the fibrin clot had been disrupted and a long junctional epithelium lined the root surface. In the demineralized specimens, the fibrin clot maintained its adhesion to the root surface and there was no apical migration of the junctional epithelium. One important result of this study was evidence that initial healing in this wound healing model tries to duplicate that seen in epidermal sites, ie, a fibrin clot does bridge the space between the two wound margins, in this case between the surgical flap and the root surface, and that initially, at least, the fibrin clot does seem to adhere

Table 3-1    Sequence of healing events at the dentin–connective tissue interface in early wound healing*

| Healing event | Observation time | | | | | |
|---|---|---|---|---|---|---|
| | 10 min | 1 h | 6 h | 1 d | 3 d | 7 d |
| Granular precipitate | X | X | X | X | X | X |
| Fibrin | X | X | X | X | X | X |
| Erythrocytes | X | X | X | X | X | X |
| Polymorphonuclear neutrophilic leukocytes | | X | X | X | X | X |
| Macrophages | | | | | X | X |
| Fibroblasts | | | | | X | X |
| Collagen | | | | | | X |

*Data gathered from light and transmission electron microscopy observations. Adapted from Wikesjö et al (1991a).

to the root surface. In addition, these observations support the concept that if this fibrin adhesion can be maintained to the root surface, there will be no apical migration of the junctional epithelium. The fibrin clot seems to block epithelial invagination into the healing wound just as it does in epidermal wounds.

More recently, Wikesjö et al (1991a) studied the early healing events at the interface of the healing wound and dentinal surfaces. Full-thickness mucoperiosteal flaps were reflected and small dentin blocks were surgically implanted into created bony concavities in edentulous alveolar ridges in two beagle dogs. The defects were created in a manner to allow a time-lapse study of initial and early healing events. Specimens for study were obtained at 10 minutes, 1 and 6 hours, and 1, 3, and 7 days after flap closure. The results were analyzed with both light and transmission electron microscopy. Healing events seemed to mirror those seen in epidermal wounds. Specimens at 10 minutes showed a granular precipitate of plasma proteins deposited on the dentin surfaces. By 1 and 6 hours there was a fibrin clot formation around red blood cell aggregates at the dentin surface. The 3-day-interval specimen showed further maturation of the fibrin clot. Macrophages were observed and for the first time fibroblasts could be identified. The 7-day specimens exhibited areas of cell-rich connective tissue replacing the fibrin clot and adhering or attached to the dentin surface as well as areas of fibrin clot in various phases of decomposition. Results are summarized in Table 3-1.

These observations confirm the earlier findings of Polson and Proye (1983) that a fibrin clot adherent to the root surface is a part of early periodontal wound healing. The results of these two studies suggest that the early period of wound healing in periodontal sites may be critical. The developing clot must form and adhere to the root surface for enough time to allow for proper wound maturation, including connective tissue formation and development, before a new connective tissue attachment to the root surface (and regeneration) can occur. Apparently, if this first series of events is disrupted, or if the initial attachment of fibrin and/or immature connective tissue is ruptured, then a pattern of healing including a long junctional epithelium is likely to occur (Polson and Proye 1983).

The importance of this "fibrin linkage" to the root surface in healing periodontal wounds was studied by Wikesjö et al (1991b), who applied heparin to the root surface to interfere with fibrin clot formation and adhesion. Heparin acts at multiple sites in the normal coagulation system to inhibit the clotting of blood and the formation of fibrin clots. It also inhibits the stabilization of the fibrin clot by inhibiting the activation of fibrin-stabilizing factors. In this study, surgical defects were created in the mandibular premolars of beagle dogs. After the defects were created, control sites were irrigated with saline and closed immediately. Experimental sites were irrigated with heparinized saline and then closed. Connective tissue reattachment to the surgically denuded root surfaces was analyzed, and heparinized and nonheparinized defects were compared histometrically. The control and experimental defects responded much differently. Nonheparinized defects healed with a mean connective tissue reattachment of 95% of the surgically created defects. Heparinized defects healed with only a mean of 50% connective tissue reattachment. The coronal 50% of the heparinized root surfaces demonstrated a marginal tissue recession of approximately 25% and a long junctional epithelium of approximately 25%. There were no statistically significant differences in the amount of bone and cementum formation between the two groups. This study seems to indicate that disruption of the fibrin clot–root surface interface leads to a healing pattern dominated by a long junctional epithelium.

The cited studies by Wikesjö et al (1991a, 1991b) and the earlier work by Polson and Proye (1983) suggest that apical migration of the gingival epithelium in periodontal wounds may not be spontaneous but may instead result from breakdown of the root surface–fibrin clot interface, thus allowing epithelial migration along the inner surface of the wound margin.

# The flap margin and its importance

The results in heparinized defects studied by Wikesjö et al (1991b) indicated substantial marginal recession, which may implicate the healing flap or wound margin as an important element in breakdown of the fibrin clot–root surface interface. During regenerative attempts, the flap (wound) margin is generally positioned so that it directly approximates the critical healing area. This margin is the area that seems most susceptible to trauma, mechanical or otherwise, which would lead to breakdown of the root surface-coagulum interface, resulting in failure of the regenerative attempt.

Klinge et al (1981, 1985), in an animal model, studied the effects of coronally positioning the flap margin to a location where it had little impact on the healing site, or stabilizing the flap by suturing it in a manner that prevented its recession and limited its movement. In the study using coronal flap displacement (Klinge et al 1981), periodontal furcation defects were surgically created in the mandibular premolars of beagle dogs. The defects were allowed to become chronic by exposure to plaque and calculus formation for 4 months after the initial surgery. They were then treated with a regenerative surgical technique including full-thickness flap elevation, root planing, and citric acid demineralization. During the regeneration attempt, flap margins were coronally positioned so that they were a mean of 4.5 mm coronal to the cemento-enamel junction (CEJ). All but the cusp tips of the teeth were covered with soft tissue (Figs 3-1a to c). Healing in the furcation area was assessed histologically. Healing was dramatically better in defects in which flap margins were coronally positioned than in defects treated in a similar manner with flap margins positioned and sutured at or near the CEJ. Nine of 15 defects treated

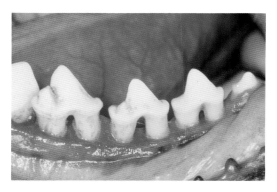

Fig 3-1a   Chronic periodontal defects in the beagle dog. Defects were created surgically 4 months previously. (Courtesy of Dr Bjorn Klinge.)

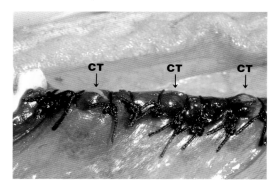

Fig 3-1b   Chronic defects treated with a coronally positioned flap procedure covering all but the cusp tips *(CT)* of the teeth.

with the coronally positioned flaps demonstrated a new connective tissue attachment in the furcations. Of 16 defects in which the flap margin was sutured at the CEJ to directly approximate the healing furcation site, one healed with a new connective tissue attachment; the other defects demonstrated an epithelized furcation.

In a second study, Klinge et al (1985) created chronic defects as previously described. Again, the regenerative surgical technique consisted of root planing and citric acid demineralization. In this study the flaps were positioned just coronal to the CEJ and were closed in the control group with interrupted interproximal sutures. In the experimental group the flap margins were positioned similarly and were closed with interproximal sutures that were bonded to the crown so that the margins were secured and stabilized in a position approximately 1 mm coronal to the CEJ until the sutures were removed after 2 weeks (see Fig 3-1). These "crown-attached" sutures prevented the flap (wound) margin from receding apically and helped to stabilize it. Histologic analysis revealed that 13 of 14 defects treated with the crown-attached sutures used to stabilize the flap margin healed with complete

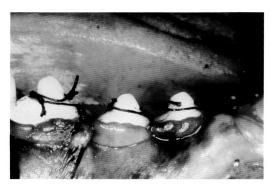

Fig 3-1c   Chronic defects treated with a crown-attached suturing technique. Flap margins are secured by sutures and bonded to the crown to limit marginal recession. (Courtesy of Dr Bjorn Klinge.)

new connective tissue attachment in the furcation itself. None of the 10 control teeth (ie, without the crown-attached sutures) showed complete new connective tissue attachment in the furcation. All demonstrated a junctional epithelium healing pattern in the furcation area. The results of these studies, as well as the previously cited work of Wikesjö et al (1991b) that showed that heparinizing surfaces induced significant marginal recession, suggest that

45

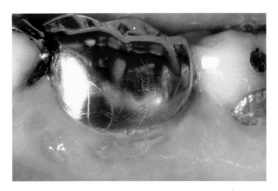

Fig 3-2a

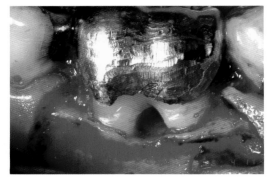

Fig 3-2b

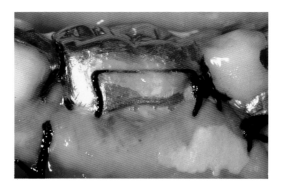

Fig 3-2c

Figs 3-2a to c   Class II mandibular molar furcation defect at the initial regenerative surgical attempt. The defect was treated with a coronally positioned flap procedure.

stability of the flap or wound margin may be important to the achievement of new connective tissue attachment and regeneration. Mobility of this margin will likely lead to tears or ruptures in the fibrin linkage to the root surface, allowing apical migration of the junctional epithelium along the inner surface of the wound, which would preclude the possibility of regeneration (Egelberg 1987).

## Current regenerative procedures

Currently the most often used regenerative techniques involve *(1)* the use of bone-inductive graft materials, *(2)* guided cell repopulation using barrier membranes, and *(3)* coronally positioned flap procedures in which the flap margin is secured an appreciable distance from the healing site. All three techniques have demonstrated clinical success, in varying degrees, in promoting periodontal regeneration and/or bone fill in periodontally diseased sites (Hancock 1989).

In terms of wound protection, these three techniques share common characteristics. Each procedure produces a space that seems necessary for a clot to form and subsequently develop into regenerated tissues. All three techniques, in differing ways, also seem to provide a means of protecting or stabilizing that clot during the early phases of healing. These areas of

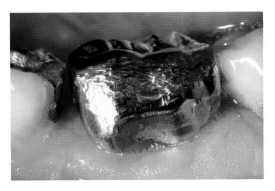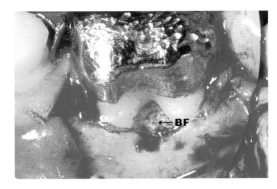

Figs 3-2d and e    Defect shown in Figs 3-2a and b at reentry 1 year after regenerative surgery. Note bone fill *(BF)* in the furcation. Figs 3-2a to e courtesy of Dr Bernard Gantes.

similarity may be as important as the traditional explanations for the effectiveness of these three procedures.

For example, the reported regenerative success of bone grafts is usually attributed to their well-documented bone-inductive properties. However, bone grafts may also serve as a scaffold for clot formation and stability and as a support for the flap itself, thus preventing early collapse of the flap into the healing wound site. This function could contribute to the successful regenerative process.

Barrier membranes, in addition to effectively eliminating gingival epithelium and gingival connective tissue from the healing wound, also seem to protect the healing clot by eliminating the effect of the flap (wound) margin on the healing site. When a membrane is placed, the root surface–wound healing interface is separated from the flap margin. The critical wound healing area is left to heal without influence from the flap margin. The barrier membrane becomes an artificial flap, which protects the healing wound. The flap margin interfaces with the barrier membrane and not with the healing wound itself. Thus, unwanted trauma or movement at the flap margin does not necessarily mean rupture of the fibrin clot–root surface interface and

breakdown that allows apical migration of the gingival epithelium.

The technique of coronally positioning and stabilizing flap margins away from the healing wound has been adapted for use in treating human mandibular class II furcation defects (Martin et al 1988). Results from two separate studies (Gantes et al 1988; Garrett et al 1990) indicate that substantial bone fill (approximately 60% to 70% of the original defect volume) can be achieved when these defects are treated with a regenerative technique that includes coronally positioning and then securing the flap margins via crown-attached sutures. In addition, when the defects were reopened a year after the initial surgery, approximately 40% to 50% of treated defects were found to have bone fill that eliminated the horizontal component of the defect. Histologic evaluation of these results to determine the amount of regeneration that has occurred awaits the obtaining of biopsy specimens, but initial results, in terms of bone fill, are encouraging (Figs 3-2a to e).

In view of the experimental evidence presented, as well as the line of reasoning discussed, the original experimental hypothesis that the prevention of apical migration of the gingival epithelium is necessary to obtain new connective tissue attachment to the root surface should perhaps be reworded into a new experimental hypothesis as suggested by Wikesjö (1991). This new hypothesis says:

1. Apical migration of the gingival epithelium in periodontal wounds is not spontaneous but results from breakdown of the root surface–fibrin clot interface.
2. Connective tissue attachment following periodontal regenerative surgery is directly related to maintenance of the root surface–adhering fibrin clot during early wound healing events.

## Future directions

There appear to be at least two important components to the dynamics of this root surface–fibrin clot interface during healing that affect the maintenance of a stable interface: tensile strength of the healing wound and biologic acceptance of the root surface.

**Tensile strength of the healing wound**

The tensile strength of the healing wound can be defined as the strength of the root surface–fibrin clot interface to resist tearing or rupture from mechanical forces (Wikesjö 1991), such as forces that mobilize the wound margin. In addition to the previously discussed methods of stabilizing the wound margin, a careful evaluation of the operative and postoperative routine applied in sites of regenerative surgery may lead to procedures that could significantly benefit the magnitude of results. If fragile tensile strength is a problem, as can be inferred from the animal studies previously discussed (Klinge et al 1981, 1985; Polson and Proye 1983; Wikesjö et al 1991b), then a postoperative routine that minimizes trauma to the wound margins during the initial phases of healing would seem important. Clinical trials are currently underway that use a postoperative routine that includes:

1. Suture materials that do not require removal until 4 to 6 weeks after the initial surgery
2. A carefully applied periodontal dressing to protect the wound during the first week of healing
3. No plaque control other than a chemotherapeutic rinse (eg, Peridex, Procter & Gamble, Cincinnati, Ohio) until 6 weeks after regenerative surgery, to avoid mechanical mobilization of the flap margins over the healing site
4. Gentle supragingival debridement of the site every 2 weeks through the first 8 weeks of healing as a means of further controlling plaque accumulation and subsequent inflammation

It will be interesting to see if minimizing potential trauma at the root surface–fibrin clot interface will produce additional beneficial results over a more conventional postoperative approach, in which little thought is given to protection of this interface.

**Biologic acceptance of the root surface**

The second and equally important component of fibrin clot adhesion to the root surface is the biologic acceptance of the root surface. Root surfaces being prepared in regenerative procedures have undergone significant changes from the norm. Conceptually, they resemble a biomaterial that needs to be altered before substantial regeneration can occur. For example, there is a phenomenon of "smear layer" postinstrumentation (Polson et al 1984). In addition, there is contamination by bacteria and bacterial products as well as endotoxins (Aleo et al 1974; Hatfield and Baumhammers 1971). Finally, along with many other factors, there is surface contamination by saliva (Heaney 1990). These changes, as well as others, may produce a surface that is biologically less than ideal for achieving and/or maintaining a stable wound healing interface. These changes may affect the tensile strength of the fibrin clot adhesion or may interfere with or alter its formation altogether.

Either or both circumstances could lead to healing via a long junctional epithelium. Attempts at improving the biologic acceptance of the root surface have consistently been a part of the regenerative literature over the past two decades. In some studies, root surfaces in periodontal defects have been partially demineralized by acid conditioning (Hancock 1989; Polson 1986). This process removes the smear layer of instrumentation, debris, blood elements, and saliva (Polson et al 1984). Partial demineralization of the root surface following thorough root planing exposes the outer layer of the collagenous matrix of dentin (Garrett et al 1978). It also removes endotoxins from the root surface (Fine et al 1980). This surface demineralization has been shown to enhance new connective tissue attachment to root surfaces in various animal models (Bogle et al 1983; Crigger et al 1978; Polson and Proye 1983). However, results in human trials have been unconvincing (Hancock 1989). In vitro studies have shown that surface demineralization of dentin surfaces will enhance the ability of these surfaces to serve as a reservoir for biologically active extracellular matrix proteins or growth factors that conceptually could alter the wound healing environment in a positive manner (Terranova and Wikesjö 1987). In addition, dentin apparently contains growth factors that may be involved in successful regeneration (Finkelman et al 1990). These could be exposed by the demineralization process.

In recent studies, extracellular matrix proteins (Alger et al 1990; Caffesse et al 1985; Smith et al 1987), polypeptide growth factors (Lynch et al 1989), and blood elements including fibronectin (Ripamonti et al 1987) have been applied to the root surface in attempts to biologically modify that surface and improve its acceptability to the cellular elements necessary to form a new connective tissue attachment. It is too premature to determine the effect of these attempts at biochemical conditioning. Results from these initial studies have varied, the vehicles to carry these biomodifiers into the healing wound have not been perfected, and the timing and concentration of their release to modify the healing response have not been determined. Yet despite these drawbacks, the biomodifiers seem to provide a potential mechanism for enhancing the regenerative capacity of healing periodontal sites.

There may be a limit to our ability to control the biomechanical factors that can affect the healing response. An accelerated healing response developed by effective use of one or a combination of potential wound healing biomodifiers may enhance regeneration beyond the present limits. It is a sobering thought to consider the unpredictability and relatively small level of regeneration achievable using today's techniques (Hancock 1989), this despite nearly three decades of attempts at regenerating the periodontium. It seems that substantial progress in this area depends on improved techniques in modifying the wound healing environment. Accelerating or enhancing the various steps in this complicated process may, in the future, prove advantageous.

## Conclusion

One aspect of the total wound healing sequence has been discussed—establishment and maintenance of the initial or early fibrin clot adhesion to the root surface. However, this is only one of a sequence of events that ends with a regenerated periodontium. Learning to control these early events so that there is a favorable outcome is just one of many steps that may be needed before substantial periodontal regeneration becomes predictable.

Over the years researchers have investigated many promising avenues that on more complete study have demonstrated equivocal success. Stabilization of the root surface–clot interface shows promise now as a necessary step to the achievement of significant regeneration. Time and experimentation will determine whether this promise will become a reality.

## Acknowledgment

Special thanks to Max Crigger, DDS, MS and Ulf Wikesjö, DDS, PhD, for their thoughtful reviews of this manuscript. Note: Since the completion of this paper, an excellent review on this subject has been published. Interested readers are referred to: Wikesjö UME, Nilveus RE, Selvig KA. Significance of early healing events on periodontal repair: A review. *J Periodontol* 1992;63:158–165.

## References

Aleo JJ, De Renzis FA, Farber PA, Varboncoeur AP. The presence and biologic activity of cementum-bound endotoxin. *J Periodontol* 1974;45:672–675.

Alger FA, Solt CW, Vuddhakanok S, Miles K. The histologic evaluation of new attachment in periodontally diseased roots treated with tetracycline-hydrochloride and fibronectin. *J Periodontol* 1990; 61:447–455.

Bogle G, Garrett S, Crigger M, Egelberg J. New connective tissue attachment in beagles with advanced natural periodontitis. *J Periodont Res* 1983;18:220–228.

Bowers GM, Chandroff B, Carnevale R, et al. Histologic evaluation of new attachment apparatus formation in humans. Part III. *J Periodontol* 1989; 60:683–693.

Caffesse RG, Holden MJ, Kon S, Nasjleti CE. The effect of citric acid and fibronectin application on healing following surgical treatment of naturally occurring periodontal disease in beagle dogs. *J Clin Periodontol* 1985;12:578–590.

Clark RAF. Overview and general considerations of wound repair. In: Clark RAF, Henson PM, eds. *The Molecular and Cellular Biology of Wound Repair.* New York: Plenum Press; 1988:3–33.

Cole RT, Crigger M, Bogle G, Egelberg J, Selvig KA. Connective tissue regeneration in periodontally diseased teeth. A histologic study. *J Periodont Res* 1980;15:1–9.

Crigger M, Bogle G, Nilvéus R, Egelberg J, Selvig KA. The effect of topical citric acid application on the healing of experimental furcation defects in dogs. *J Periodont Res* 1978;13:538–549.

Egelberg J. Regeneration and repair of periodontal tissues. *J Periodontol Res* 1987;22:233–242.

Fine DH, Morris ML, Tabak L, Cole JD. Preliminary characterization of material eluted from the roots of periodontally diseased teeth. *J Periodont Res* 1980;15:10–19.

Finkelman RD, Mohan S, Jennings JC, Taylor AK, Jepsen S, Baylink DJ. Quantitation of growth factors IGF-I, SGF/IGF-II and TGF-ß in human dentin. *J Bone Mineral Res* 1990;15:717–723.

Gantes B, Martin M, Garrett S, Egelberg J. Treatment of periodontal furcation defects. II. Bone regeneration in mandibular class II defects. *J Clin Periodontol* 1988;15:232–239.

Garrett JS, Crigger M, Egelberg J. Effects of citric acid on diseased root surfaces. *J Periodont Res* 1978;13:155–163.

Garrett S, Martin MM, Egelberg J. Treatment of periodontal furcation defects. Coronally positioned flaps versus dura mater membranes in class II defects. *J Clin Periodontol* 1990;17:179–185.

Hancock EB. Regeneration procedures. In: Nevins M, Becker W, Kornman K, eds. *Proceedings of the World Workshop in Clinical Periodontics.* Chicago: The American Academy of Periodontology; 1989: VI-1–VI-20.

Hatfield CG, Baumhammers A. Cytotoxic effects of periodontally involved surfaces of human teeth. *Arch Oral Biol* 1971;16:465–468.

Heaney TG. Inhibition of attachment of human gingival fibroblast-like cells in vitro by saliva and salivary-sulfated glycoprotein in the presence of serum. *Periodontology* 1990;61:504–509.

Klinge B, Nilvéus R, Kiger RD, Egelberg J. Effect of flap placement and defect size on healing of experimental furcation defects. *J Periodont Res* 1981;16:236–248.

Klinge B, Nilvéus R, Egelberg J. Effect of crown-attached sutures on healing of experimental furcation defects in dogs. *J Clin Periodontol* 1985;12: 369–373.

Listgarten MA, Rosenberg MM. Histological study of repair following new attachment procedures in human periodontal lesions. *J Periodontol* 1979;50: 333–344.

Lynch SE, Williams RC, Polson AM, et al. A combination of platelet-derived and insulin-like growth factors enhances periodontal regeneration. *J Clin Periodontol* 1989;16:545–548.

Martin M, Gantes B, Garrett S, Egelberg J. Treatment of periodontal furcation defects. (I) Review of the literature and description of a regenerative surgical technique. *J Clin Periodontol* 1988;15: 227–231.

Polson AM, Proye MP. Fibrin linkage. A precursor for new attachment. *J Periodontol* 1983;54:141–147.

Polson AM, Frederick GT, Landheim S, Hanes PJ. The production of a root surface smear layer by instrumentation and its removal by citric acid. *J Periodontol* 1984;55:443–446.

Polson AM. The root surface and regeneration; present therapeutic limitations and future biologic potentials. *J Clin Periodontol* 1986;13:995–999.

Ripamonti U, Petit J-C, Lemmer J, Austin JC. Regeneration of the connective tissue attachment on surgically exposed roots using a fibrin-fibronectin adhesive system. An experimental study on the baboon *(Papio ursinus). J Periodontol Res* 1987; 22:320–326.

Smith B, Caffesse R, Nasjleti C, Kon S, Castelli W. Effects of citric acid and fibronectin and laminin application in treating periodontitis. *J Clin Periodontol* 1987;14:396–402.

Steiner SS, Crigger M, Egelberg J. Connective tissue regeneration to periodontally diseased teeth. II. Histologic observations of cases following replaced flap surgery. *J Periodont Res* 1981;16:109–116.

Terranova VP, Wikesjö UME. Extracellular matrix and polypeptide growth factors as mediators of functions of cells of the periodontium. A review. *J Periodontol* 1987;58:371–380.

Wikesjö UME. *Periodontal Repair in Dogs.* Malmö, Sweden: Lund University; 1991. Thesis.

Wikesjö UME, Crigger M, Nilvéus R, Selvig KA. Early healing events at the dentin-connective tissue interface: Light and transmission electron microscopy observations. *J Periodontol* 1991a;62:5–14.

Wikesjö UME, Claffey N, Egelberg J. Periodontal repair in dogs: effect of heparin treatment of the root surface. *J Clin Periodontol* 1991b;18:60–64.

Chapter 4

# Periodontal Plastic Surgical Techniques for Regeneration

Preston D. Miller, Jr

One of the long-term desires of periodontists was to be able to cover denuded root surfaces. Beginning in the 1980s, this dream became a reality (Holbrook and Ochsenbein 1983; Miller 1982). Although marginal tissue recession seldom results in tooth loss, it is often associated with sensitivity, frenal involvements, marginal tissue irritation (because of the patient's inability or unwillingness to properly remove plaque), esthetic concerns, and a predilection to dental caries.

Some believe that if marginal tissue can be maintained free of inflammation, treatment of recession need not be considered (Dorfman et al 1980). This belief is predicated on the concept that recession is not necessarily progressive. Unfortunately, this line of thought does not take into consideration either the desires of the patient or our ability to regenerate lost oral tissue. Because root coverage procedures are quite predictable (Miller 1982) and produce patient satisfaction, it should be the therapist's obligation to make patients aware of this treatment modality.

To be considered successful, root coverage must meet the following criteria:

1. The tissue margin must be at the cementoenamel junction in class I and class II recessions.
2. The sulcus depth should be 2 mm or less.
3. There must be no bleeding on probing.
4. There should be no sensitivity.
5. The color match of the tissues should be acceptable.

Although root coverage surgery is both successful and predictable, there are still unanswered questions and concerns. First and foremost is the question of the nature of the soft tissue attachment to the root. A long junctional epithelial attachment is acceptable, but connective tissue attachment remains the treatment goal. A second concern is the role that citric acid or tetracycline might play in root biomodification. Specifically, are the root surface changes induced by acid therapy beneficial? Do they increase the predictability? Do they play a

53

role in determining the nature of the soft tissue attachment to the root? A third concern is the role barrier membranes play in root coverage (Tinti et al 1992). Last, what is the role of various growth factors in soft tissue regeneration (Terranova and Martin 1982)? The research in this area, although still in its embryonic state, offers exciting possibilities not only in osseous regeneration but also in soft tissue regeneration.

From a philosophical standpoint, root coverage procedures fit into the area of *mucogingival surgery*. However, this term, introduced in the 1950s (Friedman 1957), is dated; the process is currently known as *periodontal plastic surgery* (Miller 1988). Originally the concept of mucogingival surgery included treatment of only three defects (shallow vestibule, aberrant frenum, and inadequate attached gingiva). While periodontal plastic surgery includes treatment of those mucogingival problems, it has a much broader scope and includes surgical treatment for aberrant frena, shallow vestibules, recession (with or without root coverage), deficient ridges (ridge augmentation), maintenance of ridge form after extraction of periodontally involved teeth, excessive gingival display ("gummy smile"), unerupted teeth requiring orthodontic movement, maintenance of interdental papilla, reconstruction of lost papilla, and mucogingival defects associated with dental implants.

## Graft terminology

The terminology used in this chapter may vary from popular terminology. For example, the term *free gingival graft* will not be used. It is incorrect in two aspects. First, there is an anatomic term, *free gingival groove*, which differentiates free gingiva from attached gingiva; this free gingiva is not used in root coverage grafting. Second, *gingiva* is defined as the masticatory mucosa surrounding the teeth (American

Academy of Periodontology 1986). Palatal masticatory mucosa used in grafting is technically not gingiva because it does not surround the teeth. The ideal term, *free palatal masticatory mucosal autograft*, is not only awkward but now must be modified to include the subepithelial connective tissue graft! Therefore, the two free grafts will be described as the classic *epithelialized palatal graft* and the *subepithelial connective tissue graft*. Additionally, the term *marginal tissue recession* (Maynard and Wilson 1979) will be used rather than *gingival recession* because marginal tissue recession includes both gingival recession and alveolar mucosal recession.

## Classification of recession

Initially, marginal tissue recession was classified into four morphologic categories (Sullivan and Atkins 1968): shallow-narrow, shallow-wide, deep-narrow, and deep-wide. This classification was used from 1968 until 1985, at which time an expanded classification was presented (Miller 1985b). Root coverage can be further categorized into primary root coverage (found initially after grafting) and secondary root coverage (creeping attachment). Secondary root coverage may occur over a long period of time.

### Miller's classification

Many areas of recession fail to fall into one of the four classic categories presented by Sullivan and Atkins. Anatomic considerations, such as extruded teeth or the loss of bone or soft tissue in interproximal areas, may make it physically impossible to position the graft at the cementoenamel junction. Miller's classification addresses these anatomic considerations:

Class I   — marginal tissue recession that does not extend to the mucogingival junction. There is no periodontal loss (bone or soft tissue) in the interdental area, and 100% root coverage can be anticipated (Fig 4-1a).

Class II — marginal tissue recession that extends to or beyond the mucogingival junction. There is no periodontal loss (bone or soft tissue) in the interdental area, and 100% root coverage can be anticipated (Fig 4-1b).

Class III — marginal tissue recession that extends to or beyond the mucogingival junction. Bone or soft tissue has been lost from the interdental area, or malpositioning of the teeth prevents the attempt to achieve 100% root coverage. Partial root coverage can be anticipated (Fig 4-1c).

Class IV — marginal tissue recession that extends to or beyond the mucogingival junction. The bone or soft tissue loss in the interdental area and/or the malpositioning of the teeth is so severe that root coverage cannot be attempted (Fig 4-1d).

In class III recession, partial root coverage can be expected. The amount of root coverage can be determined presurgically with a periodontal probe. The probe is placed horizontally on an imaginary line connecting the tissue level on the midfacial surfaces of the teeth on either side of the recession. Root coverage can be anticipated to that level. If this line is marked with a pencil, the patient can graphically see the level of root coverage attainable (Fig 4-1c). The cementoenamel junction should also be outlined interdentally when there is interdental recession so that the patient can better understand the limitations of treatment.

Clinically, different classes of recession may be found on adjacent teeth. For example, one mandibular incisor may exhibit class II recession while the adjacent central incisor may exhibit class I recession. If partial root coverage is planned, instrumentation coronal to the proposed graft margin only increases and prolongs root sensitivity.

## The effect of smoking on root coverage

Surgeons have long been aware that smoking negatively affects tissue in general and healing in particular. Clinically, tissue tone and color improve when patients quit smoking.

Generally, complete root coverage cannot be attained with the epithelialized palatal graft in the smoker (Miller 1985a). Tissue alterations caused by smoking do not appear to be a factor because root coverage is attainable if patients will stop smoking immediately before the surgery and not smoke for 3 weeks after surgery.

Smoking impairs circulation (Baab and Oberg 1987) by constricting vessels and thus reducing blood flow to the graft site. In the smoker, that portion of the graft on the avascular root surface will generally slough. The subepithelial connective tissue graft offers a greater hope for root coverage in the smoker than does the epithelialized palatal graft because the former is thinner and has a blood supply to two surfaces rather than one. Coronally positioned flaps and laterally positioned pedicle grafts, although probably compromised by smoking, are not as compromised as the free grafts because they have their own blood supply. It is imperative that the surgeons point out the negative effects of smoking on any periodontal surgical procedure, especially on grafting for root coverage.

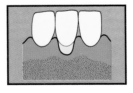 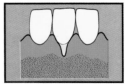 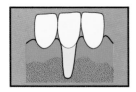 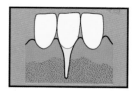

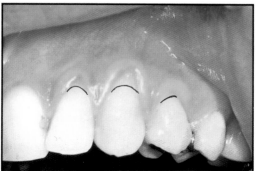 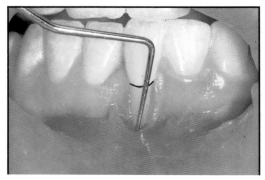

Figs 4-1a to d   From Miller 1985b. Reprinted with permission.

Fig 4-1a   Class I recession. Marginal tissue recession that does not extend to the mucogingival junction. There is no periodontal loss (bone or soft tissue) in the interdental area, and 100% root coverage can be anticipated.

Fig 4-1b   Class II recession. Marginal tissue recession that extends to or beyond the mucogingival junction. There is no periodontal loss (bone or soft tissue) in the interdental area, and 100% root coverage can be anticipated.

# Root biomodification in root coverage

Exactly how roots should be modified before root coverage procedures are attempted has never been established. The longer the roots have been exposed to bacteria and oral fluids, the more surface changes (Selvig and Zander 1962) will occur, and this could impact root biomodifications. Root biomodification may be mechanical or chemical or a combination of the two.

## Mechanical biomodification

Mechanical biomodification in its simplest form involves scaling and root planing. This may include removal of cementum, removal of softened dentin, or the smooth-

ing of surface irregularities. In more involved cases, mechanical biomodification may involve the use of rotary instruments to remove deep grooves caused by abrasion or the removal of restorations.

In using the epithelialized palatal graft for root coverage, Miller (1982) advocated flattening the root mechanically with hand instruments, especially at the cementoenamel junction. He felt this enhanced the "fit" of the butt joint margin of the graft with the cementoenamel junction. Holbrook and Ochsenbein (1983) also advocated flattening the root but for a different reason. They believed that this procedure reduced the surface area of the root mesiodistally and thus decreased the overall surface area of the avascular root that required covering. Currently, neither is a reason for exaggerated root reduction.

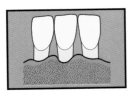
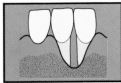
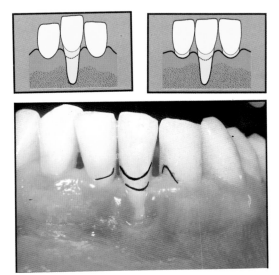
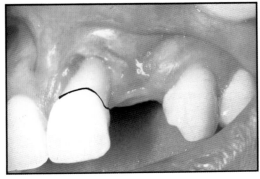

Fig 4-1c   Class III recession. Marginal tissue recession that extends to or beyond the mucogingival junction. Bone or soft tissue has been lost from the interdental area, or malpositioning of the teeth prevents the attempt to achieve 100% root coverage. Partial root coverage can be anticipated.

Fig 4-1d   Class IV recession. Marginal tissue recession that extends to or beyond the mucogingival junction. The bone or soft tissue loss in the interdental area and/or malpositioning of the teeth is so severe that root coverage cannot be anticipated.

## Chemical biomodification

Chemical biomodification has centered on acid therapy. Acid therapy, although controversial, has centered on citric acid and tetracycline hydrochloride. Although citric acid has been used clinically for more than 15 years, tetracycline has been used only recently. A lingering antimicrobial action (substantivity) and enhanced cell attachment to tetracycline-treated root surfaces are often mentioned as reasons for selecting tetracycline instead of citric acid (Frantz and Polson 1988). Unfortunately, tetracycline has also been shown to inhibit cell function (Frantz and Polson 1988). In animals, the changes produced on root surfaces by citric acid with subsequent connective tissue attachment are well documented (Bogle et al 1981)

(Figs 4-2a to i). The results in humans, however, remain controversial (Cole et al 1980; Stahl and Froum 1977). Isolated instances of connective tissue attachment have been reported following citric acid in humans, but there are no reports that tetracycline has produced a connective tissue attachment.

In a recent study, citric acid and tetracycline were compared as root conditioners (LaBahn et al 1992). Citric acid produced a greater increase in the diameter of dentinal tubules than did tetracycline. The morphologic changes produced by a 4-minute application of tetracycline could be obtained with citric acid in only 30 seconds to 1 minute. Given the data in these studies, the use of citric acid would appear to be preferable to the use of tetracycline in root biomodification.

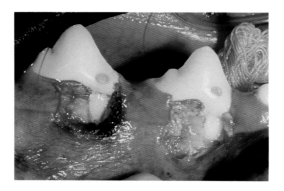

Fig 4-2a   An experimental tooth (treated with citric acid). Note the notch cut with a No. 1/2 round bur at the cementoenamel junction and the second notch cut at the apical margin of the surgically created recession.

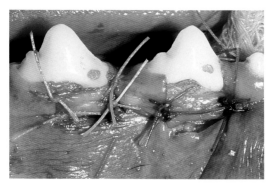

Fig 4-2b   Control tooth (non–citric acid–treated). Epithelialized soft tissue grafts were sutured at the cementoenamel junction.

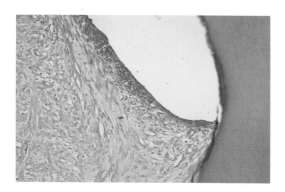

Fig 4-2c   High-power view of the notch at the cementoenamel junction of the citric acid–treated root. Note noninflammed sulcular epithelium.

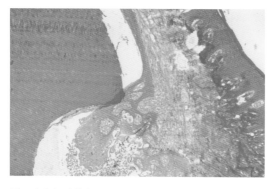

Fig 4-2d   High-power view of the notch at the cementoenamel junction of the citric acid–treated root. Note inflammatory response and epithelial migration.

Although acid therapy was used in the 19th century, Register and Burdick (1975) are credited with the revival of this technique. Having tested several acids, including citric acid and hydrochloric acid, they concluded that citric acid was the most effective and least toxic of all the acids tested. In animals they noted widening of the orifice of dentinal tubules (creating a "blunderbuss" effect) and on healing cementum formed within these tubules. They

referred to this cementum as "cementum pins" (Fig 4-2i).

Register and Burdick (1975) speculated that these "cementum pins" may form a mechanical or molecular attachment that is possibly stronger than a normal connective tissue attachment. They further speculated that citric acid may expose the collagen fibrils in the root surface and that these fibrils may "splice" with the collagen fibrils in a flap or graft. Other researchers have

Fig 4-2e *(Left)* Low-power view showing both cementoenamel junction notch and apical notch on the citric acid—treated root. Note that sulcular epithelium stops and there is no epithelial migration 7 weeks postoperatively.

Fig 4-2f *(Right)* Low-power view of the non—citric acid–treated root. Note the epithelial migration to the apical notch (7 weeks postoperatively).

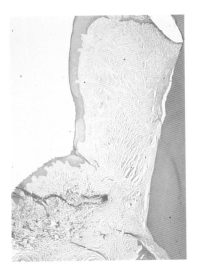 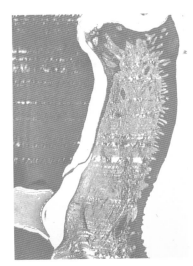

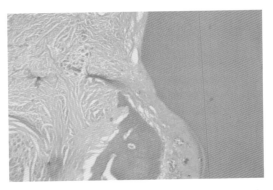

Fig 4-2g High-power view of the apical notch in the citric acid–treated root. Note the absence of epithelium and early bone formation (7 weeks postoperatively).

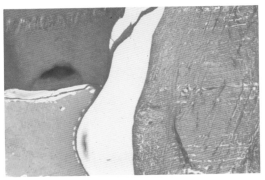

Fig 4-2h High-power view of the apical notch in the non—citric acid–treated tooth. Note the separation of soft tissue from the root, the presence of epithelium in the notch and the absence of bone formation (7 weeks postoperatively).

Fig 4-2i High-power view of the citric acid–treated root showing absence of epithelium, widening of dental tubules, cementoid formation, and cementum pins.

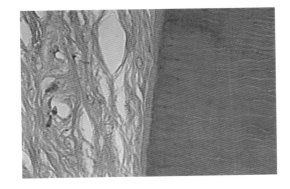

given credibility to the theory of "collagen splicing" (Codelli et al 1991). Register and Burdick (1976) further noted accelerated healing and accelerated cementogenesis as well as a connective tissue attachment when citric acid was used. Their technique included rubbing the roots with pH 1 citric acid for 3 minutes. Current research indicates that rubbing or burnishing with citric acid may not be necessary (Codelli et al 1991; LaBahn et al 1992).

Citric acid has been found to remove the "smear layer" normally found after root planing (Polson and Proye 1982). The smear layer, which is a crystalline debris layer, may interfere with attachment. Early on, fear of pulpal changes proved unfounded because citric acid produced root surface changes only a few microns deep. While citric acid may precipitate root resorption in animals, this has never been reported in humans, either experimentally or clinically.

Citric acid may demineralize subclinical bits of residual calculus left after root planing (Tanaka et al 1989). Additionally, the removal of residual endotoxins by citric acid may produce a root more amenable to attachment.

Currently no negative effects have been demonstrated in humans when roots have been treated with citric acid. By the same token, the effects on root surfaces and ultimately on healing are well documented and can be summarized as follows:

> Citric acid has been shown to remove the smear layer found on dentin surfaces following instrumentation and may open dentinal tubules, thus allowing cementum to form within these tubules and produce cementum pins. This could be associated with accelerated cementogenesis. Citric acid has also been shown to expose collagen fibrils on the root surface, which may splice with the collagen fibrils of a soft tissue graft or flap (collagen splicing), perhaps resulting in collagen adhesion without cementum formation and accelerated healing. Healing may take place at such an accelerated pace that either a connective tissue attachment or a collagen adhesion may occur before epithelium migrates, thus indirectly preventing epithelial migration. Finally, citric acid may demineralize small bits of residual calculus, disinfect the root surface, and aid in removing endotoxins.

This statement represents a summation of research findings reported in the periodontal literature over a period of nearly 20 years.

# The laterally positioned pedicle graft

The procedure currently known as the *laterally positioned pedicle graft* (Figs 4-3a to c) was originally called the *lateral sliding flap* (Grupe and Warren 1956). In this procedure, lateral gingiva is freed by a single horizontal incision and two vertical incisions and is transferred to the recipient tooth. Because this can cause recession on the donor tooth, the procedure was later modified so that a "collar" of gingiva remained on the donor tooth (Grupe 1966) (Fig 4-3a). For nearly 25 years this was the only surgical procedure available that could predictably produce coverage. The laterally positioned pedicle graft, however, has certain limitations that contraindicate its use:

1. Insufficient gingiva lateral to the recession
2. A shallow vestibule
3. Secondary frenal attachment(s) at the donor site
4. Multiple adjacent recessions

Variations of the laterally positioned pedicle graft include the double papilla

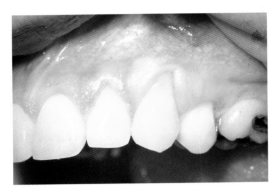

Fig 4-3a   Preoperative view of a 43-year-old woman with a 3-mm class II recession on a maxillary canine.

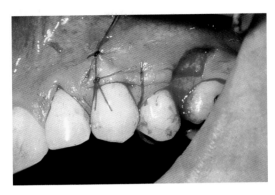

Fig 4-3b   Laterally positioned pedicle graft has been sutured. The donor site is in an interproximal area and not over a root prominence.

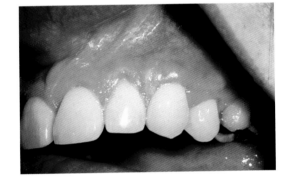

Fig 4-3c   Two-week postoperative view shows complete root coverage and excellent color match of tissue. Note the level of tissue maturity 3 weeks postoperatively.

graft (Cohen and Ross 1968) and the oblique rotated graft (Pennel et al 1965). These two procedures evolved in an attempt to use minimal amounts of gingiva for root coverage. Because other techniques for root coverage are readily available, the laterally positioned pedicle graft should only be used under ideal conditions. It thus becomes a highly predictable procedure and can create an ideal color match of tissues (Fig 4-3b).

# Epithelialized palatal graft (free gingival graft)

The classic epithelialized palatal graft was originally presented (King and Pennel 1964) as a gingival augmentation procedure with the following treatment goals:

1. To establish a soft tissue margin of keratinized tissue.
2. To prevent further recession.

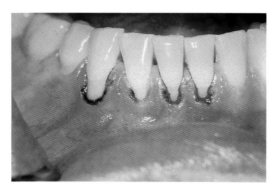

Fig 4-4a  Preoperative view of a 32-year-old man with multiple class I or early class II recessions on mandibular incisors and canine. Appearance of the roots after biomodification, which included root planing to remove residual cementum. Citric acid was burnished into the roots until the roots took on a matte finish as well as a white "milk glass" look. The time of burnishing was less than 30 seconds.

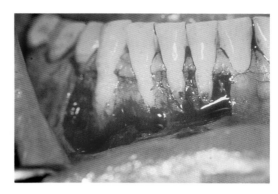

Fig 4-4b  Recipient site has been prepared with butt joint margins created in each papilla.

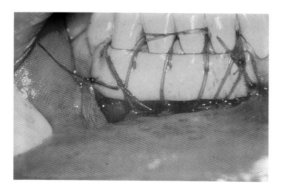

Fig 4-4c  Epithelialized palatal graft has been sutured to place with interproximal positioning sutures, apical stretching sutures, and vertical stabilizing sutures.

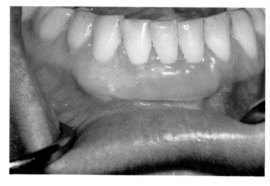

Fig 4-4d  Three-week postoperative view. Note the tissue maturity and presence of masticatory mucosa at the depth of the vestibule, which resulted in a less-than-ideal match.

3. To negate the effects of an aberrant frenum.
4. To produce a soft tissue margin that enables the patient to practice a high level of plaque removal without traumatizing the soft tissue.
5. To be an adjunctive treatment when

margins of restorations must be placed in the gingival sulcus.

Based on surgical criteria drawn from the plastic surgery literature, it was assumed that root coverage (with attachment) was not possible using the epithelialized palatal graft. However, in a study involving 100 cases, Miller (1985a) graphically demonstrated that this was not only possible but also predictable. The root coverage, while functional, unfortunately results in a graft that is readily distinguishable. On healing, the grafted palatal tissue tends to be whiter and more opaque than gingiva, and it generally extends deeper into the vestibule. The presence of grafted masticatory mucosa at the depth of the vestibule results in a match of tissues that is less than ideal (Figs 4-4a to d). Root coverage with the epithelialized palatal graft has several drawbacks:

1. The technique is difficult to perform.
2. The technique is time-consuming.
3. A blood supply to the graft is more difficult to achieve than it is for a subepithelial connective tissue graft.
4. The palatal wound (donor site) is more invasive, more prone to hemorrhage, and slower to heal. Thus it is more annoying to the patient during the healing phase.
5. The match of tissues is less than ideal.

Although the subepithelial connective tissue graft has become increasingly popular for root coverage, the epithelialized palatal graft is still used for gingival augmentation when thicker tissue is desired, when esthetics is not a concern, when there is a need to deepen the vestibule, or when pinker tissue is required as in removing an amalgam "tatoo."

## Subepithelial connective tissue graft

The subepithelial connective tissue graft represents the next stage in the evolution of free grafting for root coverage (Figs 4-5a to e). Originally presented as a ridge augmentation procedure (Langer and Calagna

1980), it was subsequently presented as a technique to be used for root coverage (Langer and Langer 1985). As a root coverage technique it offers several advantages over the epithelialized palatal graft:

1. It is not as technically demanding.
2. It is less time-consuming.
3. It is easier to establish and maintain a blood supply to the grafted tissue.
4. A palatal wound is created that is less invasive, less prone to hemorrhage, heals more rapidly, and hence is more comfortable for the patient.
5. The color match of tissues is generally better than that obtained with the epithelialized palatal graft.

Because the connective tissue is placed beneath the flap, the graft has a blood supply on two surfaces rather than a single surface. Often the recipient site can be prepared without vertical incisions by using an inverse bevel sulcular incision to create a pouch to receive the connective tissue (Fig 4-5b) (Raetzke 1985).

For root coverage, both the epithelialized palatal graft and the subepithelial connective tissue graft offer a more versatile solution than does the laterally positioned pedicle graft. With these free grafts the amount of donor tissue is not a problem and multiple recessions can be treated. Furthermore, neither a shallow vestibule nor an aberrant frenal attachment contraindicates use of these grafts.

## Coronally positioned flap

The coronally positioned flap (Figs 4-6a to c) has been used in periodontics for many years with several different variations (Harland 1907; Harvey 1965; Tarnow 1986). Although described in the early part of this century (Harland 1907), it was popularized under the term *semilunar coronal-*

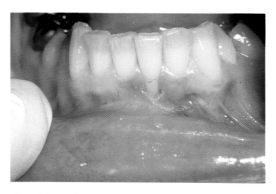

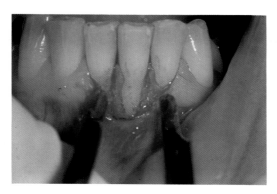

Fig 4-5a    A 54-year-old woman with class II recession on a mandibular central incisor.

Fig 4-5b    Recipient site is prepared for a connective tissue graft. There are no vertical incisions and the pouch is being held laterally with two scalpel blades for photographic purposes.

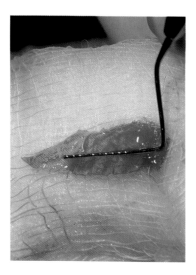

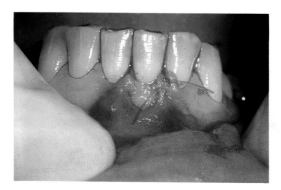

Fig 4-5c    (Left) Subepithelial connective tissue graft has been taken from the palate.

Fig 4-5d    (Above) Connective tissue graft is sutured to place. The majority of the connective tissue graft is beneath the flap, and only that portion over the denuded root is left to re-epithelialize.

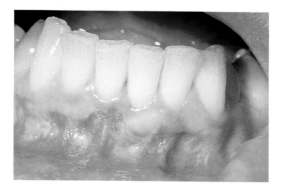

Fig 4-5e    The 18-month postoperative view shows excellent tissue match and root coverage.

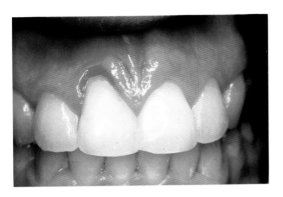

Fig 4-6a   Preoperative view of a 38-year-old woman whose maxillary central incisor exhibits recession. A "bonded" restoration was placed on the root surface; this restoration was removed during surgery.

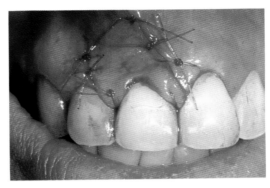

Fig 4-6b   Coronally positioned flap is sutured to place. Note the oblique incision on the mesial surface so as to avoid severing the frenum.

*ly positioned flap* (Tarnow 1986). Other researchers have presented modifications of this procedure (Allen and Miller 1989).

The procedure is limited by the height and thickness of the gingiva apical to the recession. Three millimeters of gingiva is generally believed to be the minimum height necessary if coronal positioning is to be considered. The gingiva should also be relatively thick. This procedure can only be performed on a class I recession, and if a class II or III recession is present, either a subepithelial connective tissue graft or a coronally positioned flap augmented by connective tissue should be considered.

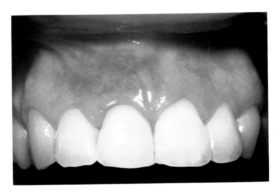

Fig 4-6c   Six-month postoperative view shows complete root coverage and excellent tissue match.

## Coronally positioned flap augmented by connective tissue

This technique has been developed by the author to meet the shortcomings of the previously mentioned coronally positioned flap, namely in the presence of an inadequate height or thickness of existing gingiva. Although this technique has been men-

tioned in the literature (Miller 1988), it has not been formally presented.

By placing connective tissue completely beneath the coronally positioned flap (gingiva or alveolar mucosa), the surgeon can produce a functional and most esthetic result (Figs 4-7a to d). If the connective tissue extends beneath the alveolar mucosa, the connective tissue on long-term healing

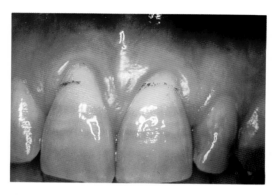

Fig 4-7a    This 27-year-old man exhibits class I recession but has very thin gingiva.

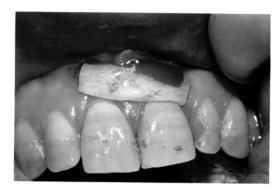

Fig 4-7b    Subepithelial connective tissue is placed under a coronally positioned flap.

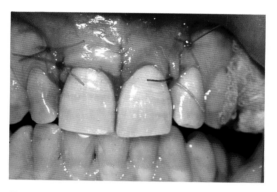

Fig 4-7c    The flap has been coronally positioned to completely cover the connective tissue.

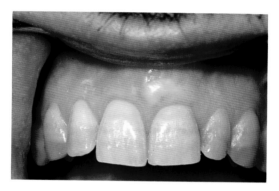

Fig 4-7d    One-year postoperative view. Note the excellent color match of tissue as well as thickness of the gingiva over both maxillary central incisors.

may become keratinized tissue (Figs 4-8a to d). In some cases the alveolar mucosa may persist but with a connective tissue base (Figs 4-9a to f). In either case, the result is functional and the esthetic tissue match is acceptable.

The surgical procedure is quite similar to the subepithelial connective tissue graft presented by Langer and Langer (1985), with one subtle difference. Rather than allowing the connective tissue to be coro-

nal to the flap, the surgeon positions the flap coronally, so that it completely covers the grafted connective tissue. Therefore, on initial healing the thickness and color match of the tissue is excellent (Fig 4-9f) because "native" tissue covers the connective tissue. When the coronal portion of a de-epithelialized subepithelial connective tissue is left exposed, the graft tends to thicken on re-epithelialization, and the esthetic result may be compromised.

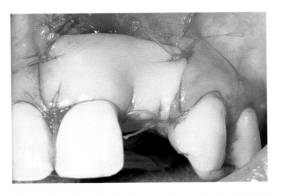

Fig 4-8a   Surgical attempt is made to create root coverage and to augment the edentulous ridge of a 48-year-old woman with a 7-mm class IV recession on two root surfaces (facial and distal).

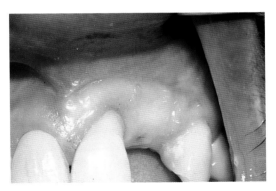

Fig 4-8b   Gingival and ridge augmentation were successful but root coverage was unsuccessful. The gingival height on the adjacent central incisor is 5 mm, but the augmented gingival height (4 mm) on the treated tooth still exhibits recession.

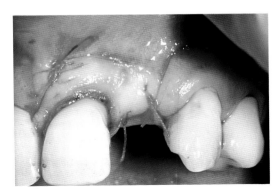

Fig 4-8c   Split-thickness coronally positioned flap has been created for root coverage (second surgical procedure). The 4-mm augmented gingiva is coronally positioned. The first 4 mm of alveolar mucosa has a connective tissue base, that is, connective tissue left by the split-thickness incision made in previously augmented gingiva.

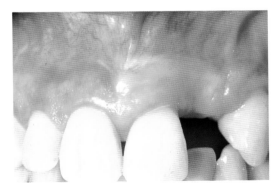

Fig 4-8d   One-year postoperative view with 8 mm of gingiva on the surgically treated central incisor. Compare the gingival height with that of the nontreated central incisor (5 mm).

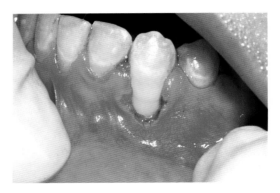

Fig 4-9a   A 19-year-old woman has a 6-mm recession and no gingiva on the facial surface of the mandibular canine.

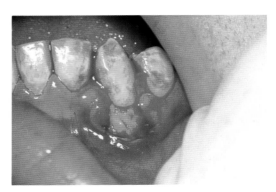

Fig 4-9b   Subepithelial connective tissue graft is placed in a "pouch" (no vertical incisions) prior to suturing. Connective tissue is still exposed.

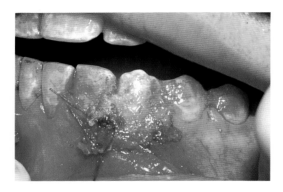

Fig 4-9c   Alveolar mucosa has been coronally positioned to completely cover the connective tissue graft. The blood clot covering the alveolar mucosa was incorporated into a surgical dressing composed of oxidized regenerated cellulose dampened with cyanoacrylate.

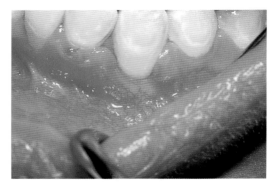

Fig 4-9d   Three-week postoperative view shows alveolar mucosa at the cementoenamel junction. The alveolar mucosa is on a connective tissue base.

## Future directions

Periodontal plastic surgery will continue to develop in direct proportion to the skilled surgeon's willingness to test innovative techniques. Today, root coverage procedures produce a more esthetic result and are simpler to perform than they were 10 years ago. This trend will continue. Although the wound incurred in harvesting palatal tissue for graft-

ing is less invasive, perhaps a future goal would be to have available a commercially produced material to substitute for subepithelial connective tissue.

Whether barrier membranes will have a place in the treatment of recession is questionable. They do appear to play a significant role in ridge augmentation. Current ridge augmentation techniques generally deal only with soft tissue augmentation

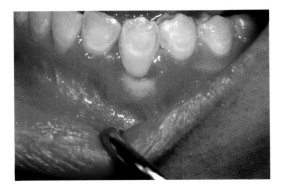

Fig 4-9e   Three-week postoperative view with tension placed on graft. Note blanching of the alveolar mucosa. The connective tissue base can be noted; the marginal tissue does not separate from the cementoenamel junction.

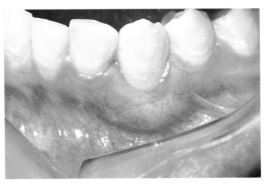

Fig 4-9f   One year postoperative view shows persistent alveolar mucosal margin but with a functional and esthetic result. Note the thickness of tissue with a connective tissue base.

and do not attempt to gain bone height. Preliminary research, however, indicates that bone fill may be attained by using barrier membranes on deficient ridges.

Growth factors appear to offer the most hope for regeneration in the future. Site-specific growth factors may be targeted to stimulate gingival connective tissue cells for the treatment of recession. The development and use of these various growth factors may represent the next step in the evolution of periodontal plastic surgery, perhaps even making barrier membranes obsolete.

# References

Allen EP, Miller PD. Coronal positioning of existing gingiva: short term results in the treatment of shallow marginal tissue recession. J Periodontol 1989; 60:316.

American Academy of Periodontology. Glossary of periodontic terms. J Periodontol 1986;57(suppl):28.

Baab D, Oberg P. Effect of cigarette smoking on gingival blood flow in humans. J Clin Periodontol 1987;14:418.

Bogle G, Adams D, Crigger M, Klinge B, Egelberg J. New attachment after surgical treatment and acid conditioning of roots in naturally occurring periodontal disease in dogs. J Periodont Res 1981; 16:130–133.

Codelli GR, Fry HR, Davis JW. Burnished versus non-burnished application of citric acid to human diseased root surfaces: the effect of time and method of application. Quintessence Int 1991;22:277–283.

Cohen DW, Ross SE. The double papillae repositioned flap in periodontal therapy. J Periodontol 1968;39:65.

Cole R, Crigger M, Bogle G, Egelberg J, Selving K. Connective tissue regeneration to periodontally diseased teeth. J Periodont Res 1980;15:1–9.

Dorfman HS, Kennedy JE, Bird WC. Longitudinal evaluation of free autogenous gingival grafts. J Clin Periodontol 1980;7:316–324.

Frantz B, Polson AM. Tissue interactions with dentin specimens after demineralization using tetracycline. J Periodontol 1988;59:714–721.

Friedman N. Mucogingival surgery. Tex Dent J 1957;75:358–362.

Grupe HE, Warren RF Jr. Repair of gingival defects by a sliding flap operation. J Periodontol 1956; 290–295.

Grupe HE. Modified technique for the sliding flap operation. J Periodontol 1966;37:491.

Harland AW. Discussion of paper: restoration of the gum tissue. Dental Cosmos 1907;49:591–598.

Harvey PM. Management of advanced periodontitis. Part I—Preliminary report of a method of surgical reconstruction. N Z Dent J 1965;61:180–187.

Holbrook T, Ochsenbein C. Complete coverage of the denuded root surface with a one-stage gingival graft. Int J Periodont Rest Dent 1983;3(3):8–27.

King KO, Pennel BM. Evaluation of attempts to increase the width of attached gingiva. Presented to the Philadelphia Society of Periodontology; 1964.

LaBahn R, Fahrenbach WH, Clark SM, Lie T, Adams DF. Citric acid and tetracycline HCL conditioning of root dentin. J Periodontol 1992;63:303–309.

Langer B, Calagna L. The subepithelial connective tissue graft. *J Prosthet Dent* 1980;44:363.

Langer B, Langer L. Subepithelial connective tissue graft technique for root coverage. *J Periodontol* 1985;56:715–720.

Maynard JG, Wilson RD. Attached gingiva and its clinical significance in the diagnosis and treatment of periodontal disease in general dental practice. In: Prichard JF (ed). The Diagnosis and Treatment of Periodontal Disease in General Dental Practice. Philadelphia: WB Saunders Co, 1979:138.

Miller PD. Root coverage using a free soft tissue autograft following citric acid application. Part I: Technique. *Int J Periodont Rest Dent* 1982;2(2):65–70.

Miller PD. Root coverage using the free soft tissue autograft following citric acid application. Part III: A successful and predictable procedure in areas of deep-wide recession. *Int J Periodont Rest Dent* 1985a;5(2):24–37.

Miller PD. A classification of marginal tissue recession. *Int J Periodont Rest Dent* 1985b;5(2):8–13.

Miller PD. Regenerative and reconstructive periodontal plastic surgery. *Dent Clin North Am* 1988;32:287–306.

Pennel BM, Higgason JD, Towner JD, King KO, Fritz BD, Salder JF. Oblique rotated flap. *J Periodontol* 1965;36:305–309.

Polson A, Proye M. Effect of root surface alterations on periodontal healing. Part II. Citric acid treatment of the denuded root. *J Clin Periodontol* 1982;9:441–454.

Raetzke P. Covering localized carious root exposure employing the "envelope technique." *J Perio* 1985;56:397–402.

Register A, Burdick F. Accelerated reattachment with cementogenesis to dentin, demineralized in situ. I. Optimum range. *J Periodontol* 1975;46:646–655.

Register A, Burdick F. Accelerated reattachment with cementogenesis to dentin, demineralized in situ. II. Defect repair. *J Periodontol* 1976;47:497–505.

Selvig KA, Zander HA. Chemical analysis and microradiography of cementum and dentin from periodontally diseased human teeth. *J Periodontol* 1962;33:303–310.

Stahl SS, Froum SJ. Human clinical and histologic repair response following use of citric acid in periodontal therapy. 1977;48:261–266.

Sullivan H, Atkins J. Free autogenous gingival grafts. III. Utilization of grafts in the treatment of gingival recession. *Periodontics* 1968;6:152–160.

Tanaka K, O'Leary T, Kafrawy A. The effect of citric acid on retained plaque and calculus. A short communication. *J Periodontol* 1989;60:81–83.

Tarnow DP. Semilunar coronally positioned flap. *J Clin Periodontol* 1986;13:182.

Terranova VP, Martin GR. Molecular factors determining gingival tissue interaction with tooth structure. *J Periodont Res* 1982;17:530–533.

Tinti C, Vincenzi G, Cortellini P, Pini Prato GP, Clauser C. Guided tissue regeneration in the treatment of human facial recession. A 12-case report. *J Periodontol* 1992;63:554–560.

# Chapter 5

# Osseous Grafts and Periodontal Regeneration

James T. Mellonig

Freeze-dried bone allografts were introduced to periodontics in the early 1970s but had been used in orthopedic medicine since 1950. The development of periodontal bone allografts as an alternative source of graft material was spurred by the disadvantages of autogenous bone. This included the need for a secondary surgical site to procure donor material and the frequent lack of intraoral donor sites to obtain sufficient quantities of autogenous bone for multiple or deep osseous defects. The added disadvantages of fresh frozen bone allografts, namely the possibility of disease transfer, immunogenicity, and the need for cross matching (Schallhorn 1977), made freeze-dried bone allografts even more attractive because they are devoid of these limitations. Today, freeze-dried bone allografts are used routinely in periodontal therapy. It is estimated that more than 40,000 bottles of freeze-dried bone allograft are used annually for dental purposes. This chapter will discuss the studies conducted at the Navy Dental School, Bethesda, Maryland, in the development of periodontal freeze-dried bone allografts, and the

current status and future directions of such allografts.

## Field test studies

In 1972, a field test study was initiated to evaluate the potential of undemineralized cortical freeze-dried bone allograft (FDBA) as a periodontal graft material. Eighty-nine clinicians throughout the United States were invited to participate as collaborators. They were asked to evaluate this graft material in all types of intraosseous defects including furcations. Each clinician was given the option of flap design, fill or overfill of the defect, antibiotic regimen, use of a periodontal dressing, and whether or not to perform intramarrow penetration of the cortical lining surrounding the osseous defect. Documentation consisted of preoperative and postoperative probing depth measurements from a fixed reference point, defect depth measurements, photographs, and radiographs. At 1 year, a surgical reentry was to be performed and all measurements were repeated. The clinician was then to determine the extent of

**Table 5-1**  Clinical evaluation of freeze-dried bone allograft; hard tissue results following surgical reentry

| Defect type | n | Bone fill | | | |
|---|---|---|---|---|---|
| | | Complete | > 50% | < 50% | Failed |
| 1-walled | 53 | 19 | 18 | 12 | 4 |
| 2-walled | 70 | 21 | 32 | 12 | 5 |
| 3-walled | 38 | 6 | 24 | 6 | 2 |
| 1-2-walled | 49 | 10 | 21 | 13 | 5 |
| 1-3-walled | 26 | 5 | 12 | 8 | 1 |
| 2-3-walled | 50 | 7 | 26 | 12 | 5 |
| Furca | 43 | 10 | 9 | 4 | 20 |
| | | | | | |
| *Total* | *329* | *78* | *142* | *67* | *42* |
| | | (24%) | (43%) | (20%) | (13%) |
| | | | 220 | | 109 |
| | | | (67%) | | (33%) |

**Table 5-2**  Clinical evaluation of freeze-dried bone allograft; soft tissue results

| Defect type | n | Probing depth reduction | | | |
|---|---|---|---|---|---|
| | | Complete | > 50% | < 50% | Failed |
| 1-walled | 53 | 19 | 17 | 13 | 4 |
| 2-walled | 69 | 20 | 29 | 16 | 4 |
| 3-walled | 37 | 7 | 21 | 7 | 2 |
| 1-2-walled | 49 | 15 | 20 | 11 | 3 |
| 1-3-walled | 26 | 6 | 14 | 6 | 0 |
| 2-3-walled | 50 | 11 | 27 | 10 | 2 |
| Furca | 43 | 9 | 10 | 10 | 14 |
| | | | | | |
| *Total* | *327* | *87* | *138* | *73* | *29* |
| | | (27%) | (42%) | (22%) | (9%) |
| | | | 225 | | 102 |
| | | | (69%) | | (31%) |

probing depth reduction and bone fill of the defect as complete, greater than 50%, less than 50%, or failure.

A total of 997 sites were implanted with FDBA alone and 524 by a composite graft technique of FDBA plus autogenous bone (FDBA + A). Sufficient data, as determined by surgical reentry of the defect site at 6 months or longer postoperatively, were collected to determine success or failure in 329 sites treated with FDBA and 176 sites treated with FDBA + A (Tables 5-1 to 5-4). The result of greater than 50% or complete bone fill in 67% of the sites treated confirmed the early findings of 64%, 60%, and 63% (Mellonig et al 1976; Sepe et al 1978; Sanders et al 1983). Likewise, a probing depth reduction of 69% confirmed earlier findings of 70%, 63%, and 65%. Augmentation of the FDBA with autogenous bone enhanced bone fill, especially in furcation defects (Figs 5-1a to c). Seventy-eight of

**Table 5-3**  Clinical evaluation of freeze-dried bone allograft plus autogenous bone; hard tissue results following surgical reentry

| Defect type | n | Bone fill | | | |
|---|---|---|---|---|---|
| | | Complete | > 50% | < 50% | Failed |
| 1-walled | 23 | 5 | 12 | 5 | 1 |
| 2-walled | 32 | 12 | 16 | 3 | 1 |
| 3-walled | 46 | 10 | 26 | 3 | 7 |
| 1-2-walled | 17 | 8 | 4 | 3 | 2 |
| 1-3-walled | 3 | 1 | 1 | 0 | 1 |
| 2-3-walled | 38 | 9 | 18 | 8 | 3 |
| Furca | 17 | 6 | 9 | 2 | 0 |
| *Total* | *176* | *51* | *86* | *24* | *15* |
| | | (29%) | (49%) | (14%) | (8%) |
| | | | 137 | | 39 |
| | | | (78%) | | (22%) |

**Table 5-4**  Clinical evaluation of freeze-dried bone allograft plus autogenous bone; soft tissue results

| Defect type | n | Probing depth reduction | | | |
|---|---|---|---|---|---|
| | | Complete | > 50% | < 50% | Failed |
| 1-walled | 23 | 6 | 14 | 2 | 1 |
| 2-walled | 32 | 14 | 13 | 5 | 0 |
| 3-walled | 46 | 14 | 19 | 0 | 7 |
| 1-2-walled | 17 | 7 | 3 | 3 | 1 |
| 1-3-walled | 3 | 1 | 1 | 1 | 0 |
| 2-3-walled | 38 | 11 | 16 | 7 | 4 |
| Furca | 15 | 8 | 6 | 1 | 0 |
| *Total* | *174* | *63* | *75* | *24* | *12* |
| | | (36%) | (43%) | (14%) | (7%) |
| | | | 138 | | 36 |
| | | | (78%) | | (21%) |

the defects treated responded with complete or greater than 50% bone fill.

Analysis of the clinical parameters indicated that the number of osseous walls lining the defect, intramarrow penetration, prior endodontic therapy, and flap type had no statistical bearing on success or failure. Only the use of antibiotics and type of flap closure positively affected success or failure. Tetracycline was the most frequently used antibiotic.

Freeze-dried bone allograft alone was more efficacious in the treatment of intra-osseous or walled defects than furcation lesions, but results in these defects were not statistically different when the composite FDBA + A was used. The possibility that operator experience or total procedures performed might affect success and failure was evaluated. These factors were found not to have any influence on treatment results.

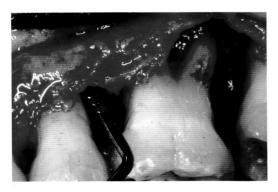

Fig 5-1a   Class II furcation involvement on a maxillary first molar with a deep intraosseous defect on the mesial surface.

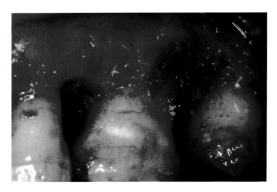

Fig 5-1b   Freeze-dried bone allograft plus an autogenous bone graft implanted into the defects.

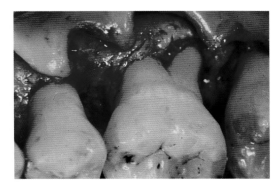

Fig 5-1c   Complete to greater than 50% noted at a 1-year reentry.

# Regeneration of the periodontium with FDBA

To test if regeneration of a new attachment apparatus were possible following a graft of FDBA, periodontal osseous defects were grafted in adult male baboons (Mellonig 1981). Orthodontic elastic bands were placed bilaterally on alternate posterior teeth and allowed to migrate subgingivally (Caton and Kowalski 1976). At the end of 7 to 9 months, the elastic bands were removed. An additional 3 months was allowed to elapse to ensure that the defects were nonhealing. Sixty angular bone defects (30 matched pairs) of approximately 2 to 3 mm in depth were created in four baboons. Cortical bone from the fibula of a female adult baboon was frozen, freeze-dried, and ground to a mean particle size of 250 μm. A notch was placed in the root surface at the base of each defect. Each matched pair was either treated with an FDBA bone graft or left empty as the control (open flap debridement). The animals were killed 5 to 12 months postsurgery.

From these studies, it was concluded that grafting with FDBA alone or in combination with autogenous bone has potential in the treatment of periodontal osseous defects. If furcation lesions are to be treated, the composite graft (FDBA + A) is indicated.

As a result of this field test study, other questions arose. Was regeneration or repair of the periodontium achieved? Was FDBA antigenic in the periodontal environment?

The jaws were dissected free and fixed in formalin. Blocks containing graft and

**Table 5-5** Regeneration with freeze-dried bone allograft in periodontal osseous defects of the baboon: analysis of 60 defects

| Animal No. | Months postsurgery | FDBA | | | Control | | |
|---|---|---|---|---|---|---|---|
| | | | Regeneration | | | Regeneration | |
| | | Defects | Yes | No | Defects | Yes | No |
| 1 | 5 | 3 | 2 | 1 | 3 | 1 | 2 |
| 2 | 5 | 4 | 4 | 0 | 4 | 0 | 4 |
| 3 | 6 | 4 | 0 | 4 | 4 | 0 | 4 |
| 2 | 7 | 4 | 2 | 2 | 4 | 1 | 3 |
| 1 | 8 | 4 | 3 | 1 | 4 | 2 | 2 |
| 4 | 8 | 3 | 2 | 1 | 3 | 1 | 2 |
| 3 | 9 | 4 | 1 | 3 | 4 | 0 | 4 |
| 4 | 12 | 4 | 2 | 2 | 4 | 0 | 4 |
| *Total* | | 30 | 16 | 14 | 30 | 5 | 25 |

Chi-square with Yates correction = 7.326; *df* = 1; *P* < .01.

control sites were demineralized and mounted in a mesiodistal plane. The sections were cut at 12-μm thicknesses, and step serial sections at 96-μm intervals were mounted and stained.

Histologic analysis was performed on step serial sections at 192-μm intervals with a calibrated grid mounted in the eyepiece of a light microscope × 40. Each section was evaluated for the presence of regeneration. New bone, new cementum, and new periodontal ligament had to be present throughout the entire block for the evaluator to determine regeneration had occurred. The notch at the base of the defect was used as the histologic reference point, and linear measurements were made along the root surface to *(1)* the most apical cells of the junctional epithelium, *(2)* the most coronal aspect of new cementum, *(3)* the crest of the interproximal bone, and *(4)* the apical extent of angular bone defect.

The results demonstrated that regeneration of the attachment apparatus was present in 16 of 30 defects treated with FDBA and 5 of 25 control sites (Table 5-5). The results were also analyzed for differences

**Table 5-6** Regeneration with freeze-dried bone allograft in periodontal osseous defects of the baboon: analysis of matched-pair defects for new bone, cementum, and periodontal ligament

| Graft | Regeneration | No. of pairs |
|---|---|---|
| FDBA | Yes | 11 |
| Control | No | |
| FDBA | Yes | 5 |
| Control | Yes | |
| FDBA | No | 0 |
| Control | Yes | |
| FDBA | No | 14 |
| Control | No | |

Chi square = 9.205; *df* = 1; *P* < .01.

in matched pairs (Table 5-6). Both methods of analysis indicated that the differences were statistically significant. Histomorphometric analysis showed that more new bone, new cementum, and new periodontal ligament were present in grafted sites than nongrafted sites (Fig 5-2). These differences were likewise statistically significant in favor of using FDBA. It was concluded that the probability of obtaining

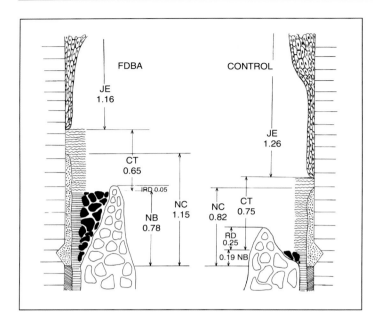

Fig 5-2  Histologic evaluation of regeneration after a freeze-dried bone allograft or open flap curettage in periodontal osseous defects of baboons. Mean serial section measurements of 60 defects (30 pairs) in millimeters. *P* < .05; paired sample *t* test. *JE* = junctional epithelium; *CT* = connective tissue attachment; *NB* = new bone formation; *NC* = new cementum formation; RD = residual defect.

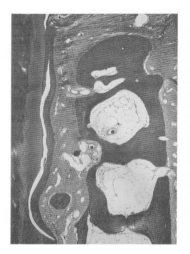 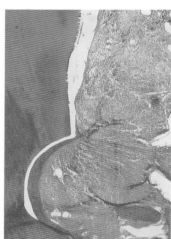 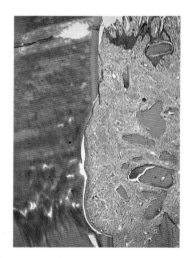

Fig 5-3  *(Left)* Section from the mesial surface of maxillary right first molar of animal no. 1, grafted with freeze-dried bone allograft, demonstrating new bone, cementum, and periodontal ligament coronal to the notch placed in cementum. (Hematoxylin and eosin stain; original magnification × 25.)

Fig 5-4  *(Middle)* Section from the mesial surface of the maxillary left first molar of animal no. 1, open flap debridement (control), demonstrating a long junctional epithelium with no regeneration. (Hematoxylin and eosin stain; original magnification × 25.)

Fig 5-5  *(Right)* Section obtained 1 month after a graft of freeze-dried bone allograft. Note new cementum and early new bone formation around graft particles.

regeneration in this model system is enhanced when FDBA is used (Figs 5-3 and 5-4). A fifth baboon served as an early wound healing model. At 1 month post-surgery, new bone and new cementum could be seen (Fig 5-5).

## Antigenicity of FDBA

Friedlaender et al (1984) demonstrated by microcytotoxicity tests that 9 of 43 patients receiving large FDBA bone grafts for treating orthopedic bone tumors developed anti-HLA antibodies. Therefore, the potential exists for a graft of FDBA in the periodontal tissues to be immunogenic. To determine if cortical bone allografts preserved by freeze drying could elicit an antigenic response, FDBA was implanted into periodontal osseous defects of both baboons and humans.

Cortical bone was removed from a donor baboon, deep frozen, and then freeze dried (Turner and Mellonig 1981). Cancellous bone and marrow were removed from the same donor animal. A mixed lymphocyte culture indicated incompatibility in the case of both donor and recipient baboons and was predictive of allograft rejection.

Angular periodontal osseous defects were created in three recipient baboons. Two received grafts of FDBA and the third a graft of fresh cancellous bone and marrow allograft. Three months later the animals received a second set of identical grafts. Microcytotoxicity assays were used as a measure of both humoral and cell-mediated immunity. The results indicated that there was markedly less humoral and cell-mediated immune response to freeze-dried cortical bone allografts in comparison to fresh bone grafts.

The next objective was to determine whether donor-specific anti-HLA antibodies could be detected against FDBA implanted in human periodontal osseous defects (Quattlebaum et al 1988). Twenty patients with multiple and deep periodontal osseous defects participated in this study as recipients of FDBA. All bone was procured from one donor of known HLA tissue type. No recipient of the FDBA had preexisting anti-HLA antibodies. Serum samples were taken 2 weeks after the first allograft (primary challenge), 2 weeks after the second allograft (secondary challenge), and at 3 months. Serum samples were assayed for the presence of anti-HLA antibodies using an Amos-modified microcytotoxicity assay. At no time could any donor-specific anti-HLA antibodies be detected in any patient. All FDBA grafts were judged to be clinically successful. No adverse reaction was noted.

From these studies it was concluded that periodontal bone grafts of FDBA have a markedly reduced antigenicity. This conclusion is consistent with the long history of clinical safety associated wth allografts of freeze-dried cortical bone. The freeze-drying process may spatially distort the three-dimensional presentation of HLA antigens on FDBA, affecting immune recognition (Friedlaender et al 1984).

## Comparison of bone graft materials

The thrust of the next several studies was to determine how FDBA compares with other bone graft materials in its ability to induce new bone formation. The bone-forming abilities of autogenous osseous coagulum, autogenous bone blend, freeze-dried bone allograft (FDBA), and decalcified freeze-dried bone allograft (DFDBA) were compared.

Intraoral cortical bone, when obtained with high- or low-speed burs and mixed

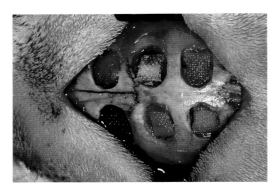

Fig 5-6a  Graft materials within nylon chambers inserted into calvaria defects. One implant chamber remains empty to serve as the control. An additional defect receives no implant.

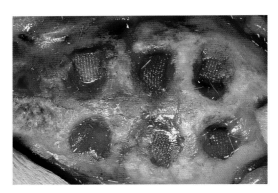

Fig 5-6b  Graft materials within nylon chambers prior to removal at 21 days postimplantation. Note wound healing.

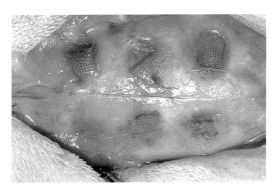

Fig 5-6c  Graft materials prior to removal from defect site at 42 days postinsertion.

with the patient's blood, becomes a coagulum (Robinson 1969). The rationale for the use of osseous coagulum is based on the beliefs that the smaller the particle size of donor bone, the more certain are its resorption and replacement with host bone, and that mineralized fragments can induce bone formation. Case reports indicate that intraosseous defects can be successfully managed with this graft material (Robinson 1969).

Bone blend is cortical or cancellous intraoral bone that is procured with a trephine bur or rongeurs, placed in an amalgam capsule, and triturated to the consistency of a "slushy" osseous mass (Diem et al 1972). A mean bone fill of 73% was obtained in 25 defects (Froum et al 1975). Froum et al (1976) also reported that the osseous coagulum-bone blend graft provided 2.98 mm of coronal growth of alveolar bone, compared to 0.66 μm obtained when open flap debridement alone was used.

Urist and coworkers demonstrated through numerous animal experiments that demineralization and freeze drying of a cortical bone graft induce new bone formation and greatly enhance its osteogenic potential (Urist 1965; Urist et al 1967, 1968, 1975). Demineralization was thought to be necessary because the bone mineral blocked the effect of the chemical inductive agent (Urist and Strates 1970). This chemical component of the bone matrix was termed *bone morphogenetic protein* (BMP) (Urist and Strates 1971). Bone morphogenetic protein is composed of a group of acidin polypeptides that have been cloned and sequenced (Urist et al 1983; Wozney et al 1988). It stimulates the formation of new bone by osteoinduction (Urist et al 1970); that is, the DFDBA induces the host stem cells to differentiate into osteoblasts

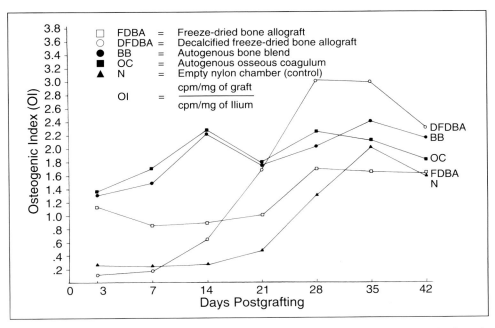

Fig 5-7 Data derived for the mean osteogenic index (rate of bone formation) of each graft preparation and the controls. Each coordinate represents five samples. The osteogenic index relates the uptake of strontium 85 into new bone evoked by the samples to the uptake in the ilium on a weight basis.

(Harakas 1984). An undemineralized allograft, such as FDBA, is thought to function by osteoconduction, because it affords a scaffold over which new bone forms (Goldberg and Stevenson 1987).

Defects were created in the calvaria of 35 guinea pigs (Mellonig et al 1981a). These defects were nonhealing. Cortical bone from the femurs of donor animals served as a source of bone allograft, and calvarial bone from recipient animals became the source for the autogenous grafts. Autogenous osseous coagulum, autogenous bone blend, DFDBA, and FDBA were inserted into porous nylon chambers and implanted into the defects (Figs 5-6a to c). Empty nylon chambers served as the controls. Three days before it was killed, each animal received an injection of strontium 85 (Sr 85). Strontium 85 selectively concentrates into immature

new bone and can be used as a measure of the rate of new bone formation (Elves 1974). The animals were killed in groups of five at 3, 7, 14, 21, 28, 35, and 42 days. A small section of ilium was removed from each animal. This served as a standard for the rate of new bone formation. The samples were recovered and weighed, and the uptake of Sr 85 into new bone was determined. An osteogenic index was obtained by dividing cpm/mg of sample by cpm/mg of ilium for each animal.

The rate of new bone formation in the presence of DFDBA increased very rapidly from day 14 to day 28 and declined thereafter. Decalcified freeze-dried bone allograft had a more rapid rate of osteogenesis than autogenous osseous coagulum, autogenous bone blend, FDBA, or the control (Fig 5-7). It was concluded that in this model system, DFDBA is a graft material

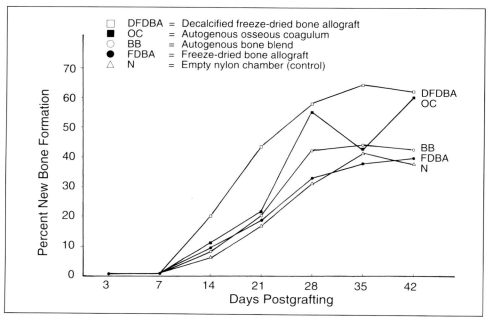

Fig 5-8   New bone formation in response to autografts and allografts in nylon chambers implanted in guinea pig calvaria. Each coordinate represents the total amount of bone formation at each study period.

of high osteogenic potential while autogenous osseous coagulum and autogenous bone blend are of less potential, and FDBA of even less. The rate of bone formation with FDBA was, however, greater than that of the control.

The same samples that were evaluated for the rate of new bone formation were now compared histologically for total amount of newly formed bone over each study period (Mellonig et al 1981b). The percent of new bone formation evoked by the graft materials and the control at various time periods is presented in Fig 5-8. At no time was the percentage of new bone induced by DFDBA less than that induced by autogenous osseous coagulum, autogenous bone blend, FDBA, or the empty nylon chamber (Figs 5-9a to e). The autogenous materials (osseous coagulum and bone blend) evoked more new bone for-

mation than FDBA. The control and FDBA paralleled each other in the percentage of new bone formed. These results confirmed the results analyzed by Sr 85.

In phase II, the same experimental design was used to evaluate composite grafts of autografts and allografts (Mellonig et al 1980). The following were compared: DFDBA plus osseous coagulum, DFDBA plus bone blend, FDBA plus osseous coagulum, and FDBA plus bone blend. A defect with an empty nylon chamber was the control, and FDBA alone was implanted to compare phase I to phase II. A single defect in each animal remained unimplanted as a measure of the healing potential of the calvarial defect. Equal amounts by volume of autograft and allograft were combined, inserted into nylon chambers, and implanted in 35 animals. The animals were killed in groups of five at weekly intervals from 3 to

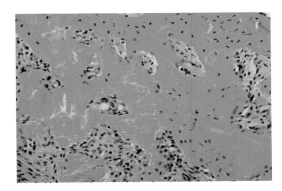

Fig 5-9a   New bone formation adjacent to particles of osseous coagulum, 21 days postgrafting. (Hematoxylin and eosin stain; original magnification × 63.)

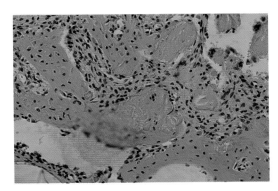

Fig 5-9b   New bone formation adjacent to particles of bone blend, 21 days postgrafting. (Hematoxylin and eosin stain; original magnification × 63.)

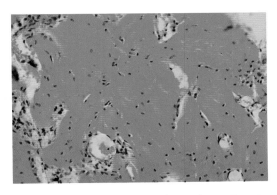

Fig 5-9c   Abundant new bone formation in direct contact and in clefts and spaces within decalcified freeze-dried bone allograft, 21 days postgrafting. (Hematoxylin and eosin stain; original magnification × 63.)

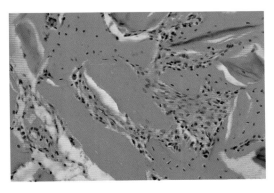

Fig 5-9d   New bone formed on particles of freeze-dried bone allograft, 21 days postgrafting. (Hematoxylin and eosin stain; original magnification × 63.)

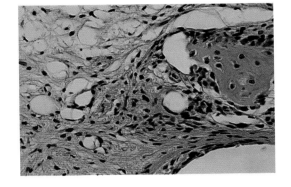

Fig 5-9e   Bone formation near border within empty control chamber. Most of the chamber is occupied by connective tissue (21 days postgrafting). (Hematoxylin and eosin stain; original magnification × 63.)

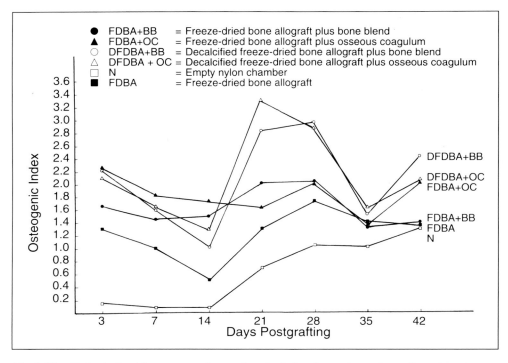

Fig 5-10  Data derived for mean osteogenic rate (rate of new bone formation at each sacrifice period) of each graft composite preparation and the controls. Each coordinate represents five samples.

42 days. Strontium 85 was injected into each animal 3 days before it was killed. Results indicated that as a group, no difference could be found in the rate of bone growth of the composite graft materials. The rate of bone growth was greater with the composite grafts than for FDBA alone, and the rate with FDBA was greater than that with the empty nylon chamber (Fig 5-10). As in phase I, the unimplanted control did not spontaneously heal over the 42-day experimental period.

New bone formation was also determined by a quantitative histologic technique for the percent of new bone (Mellonig et al 1982). Analysis for total amount of new bone formed at each time period suggested that the combination of DFDBA plus osseous coagulum or DFDBA plus bone blend has a greater osteogenic potential than composite grafts of FDBA plus osseous coagulum or FDBA plus bone blend (Fig 5-11). It was suggested from experiments conducted in phase II that composite grafts of autogenous and demineralized allogenic bone enhance new bone formation more than other graft materials.

In phase III, the osteogenic potential of autogenous marrow and composites of autogenous marrow with DFDBA and FDBA were compared (Mellonig et al 1983). The same experimental model and methods of analysis were used as in phase I and phase II of this study. As a group, there was no statistical difference

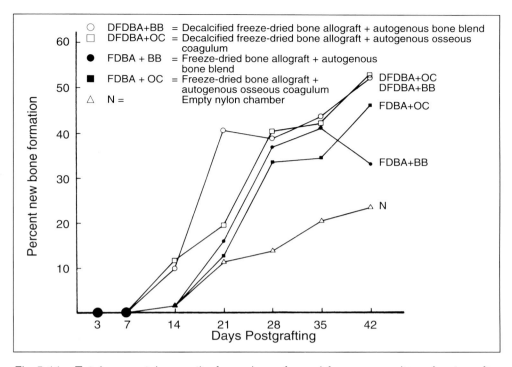

Fig 5-11   Total amount (percent) of new bone formed from composites of autografts-allografts at each time period.

between autogenous marrow, DFDBA plus marrow, or FDBA plus marrow. Autogenous marrow and the composites were greater in osteogenic potential than FDBA alone, which was greater in osteogenic potential than was the empty nylon chamber (Figs 5-12 and 5-13).

There was no statistically significant difference between the osteogenic indices for FDBA alone among phases I, II, and III. Likewise there was no statistically significant difference among the osteogenic indices of the empty nylon chambers in phases I, II, and III. Therefore the results for FDBA (Fig 5-14) and its composites and DFDBA and its composites (Fig 5-15) were compared. An osteogenic profile over the peak periods of bone formation (days

14 to 35) was developed (Fig 5-16). It was concluded that:

1. Marrow alone induces a fast rate of new bone formation.
2. Decalcified freeze-dried bone allograft is superior to FDBA as a graft material.
3. The addition of autogenous materials bone blend or osseous coagulum enhances the osteogenic potential of FDBA.
4. The addition of marrow to FDBA greatly improves its osteogenic potential.
5. The addition of autogenous bone to DFDBA to form a composite does not greatly enhance its osteogenic potential.
6. By itself, DFDBA is a potent inducer of new bone formation.

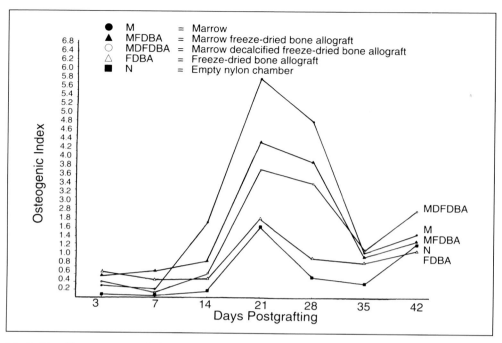

Fig 5-12   Mean osteogenic index (rate of bone formation) for marrow and allograft-marrow composites over the 3-day period from injection of Sr 85 to sacrifice.

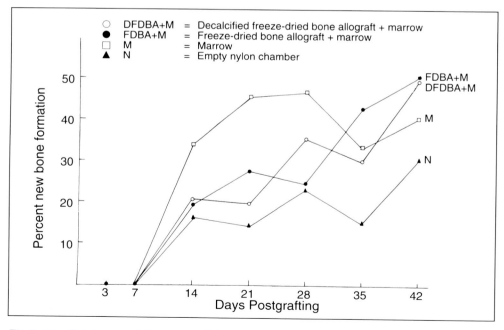

Fig 5-13   Total amount (percent) of bone formed at each study period for autogenous marrow and allograft-marrow composites.

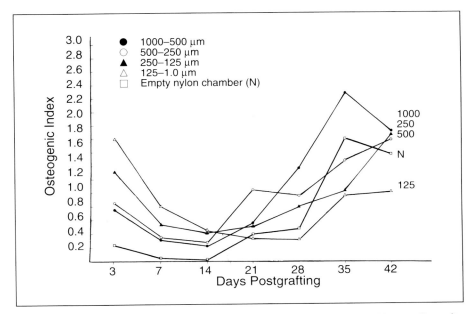

Fig 5-17   Osteogenic index of different particle sizes of freeze-dried bone allograft.

is seen with the larger particle sizes. The amount of new bone formation was also determined by quantitative histologic technique. Particle sizes in the range of 125 to 1,000 μm produce more new bone than do particles sized 125 μm and below (Figs 5-18a to d). Particle sizes in the range of 250 to 1,000 μm are also significantly better than particle sizes 250 μm and below. It was concluded that in this model system, FDBA with a particle size of 250 to 1,000 μm has a higher osteogenic potential than does FDBA with a particle size of 250 μm and below. Histologic analysis further suggests that a particle size of 125 μm and below may actually be counterproductive for osteogenesis. Based on this investigation and previously cited studies, a particle size in the range of 250 to 750 μm is recommended for periodontal bone grafting procedures. Studies also suggest that pore size is important when considering new

bone growth. A pore size in the range of 100 to 200 μm is considered optimal for endothelial and fibroblastic ingrowth (Bhaskar et al 1971; Hulbert et al 1970; Topazian et al 1971). Therefore, the space between the particles may be just as important as the size of the particles themselves.

# Decalcified freeze-dried bone allograft

### Case reports

Cortical bone was obtained under sterile conditions from the femur of a single human donor within 12 hours of death. It was defatted in chloroform-methanol, autodigested in a phosphate buffer, and

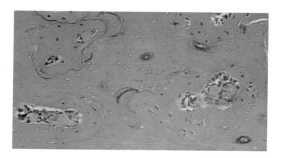

Fig 5-18a    Amount of bone formed in response to 500- to 1,000-μm particles of freeze-dried bone allograft at 35 days. (Hematoxylin and eosin stain; original magnification × 63.)

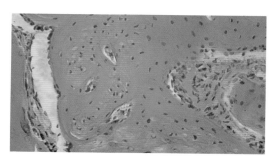

Fig 5-18b    Amount of bone formed in response to 250- to 500-μm particles of freeze-dried bone allograft at 35 days. (Hematoxylin and eosin stain; original magnification × 63.)

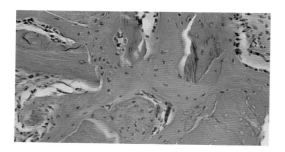

Fig 5-18c    Amount of bone formed in response to 125- to 250-μm particles of freeze-dried bone allograft at 35 days. (Hematoxylin and eosin stain; original magnification × 63.)

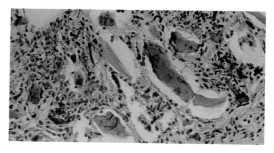

Fig 5-18d    No new bone formation with 1- to 125-μm particles of freeze-dried bone allograft. Note multinucleated giant cells. (Hematoxylin and eosin stain; original magnification × 63.)

demineralized with 0.6 sodium hydrochloride by the method of Urist et al (1975). The bone was ground to a particle size of 250 to 500 μm, frozen, and freeze dried. The cortical DFDBA was implanted into 27 one-, two- and three-walled defects of 11 patients (Quintero et al 1982). Clinical measurements were made, using the base of a stent as a fixed reference point, for gain or loss of clinical attachment. Measurements at the time of surgery were made for alveolar crest height and depth of osseous defect. All measurements were repeated at the time of a 6-month reentry.

There was an average bone fill of 2.6 mm in 5 one-walled defects, 1.8 mm in 14 two-walled defects, and 2.9 in 8 three-walled defects. This represented mean bone fills of 61%, 62%, and 73%, respectively. The overall mean for the 27 defects was 2.4 mm (65%) (Figs 5-19a to c). There

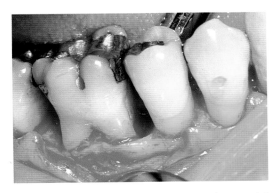

Fig 5-19a  Intraosseous defect on the mesial surface of the mandibular first molar.

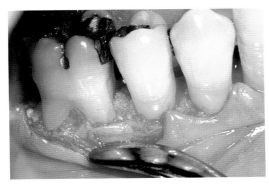

Fig 5-19b  Defect implanted with decalcified freeze-dried bone allograft; particle size is 250 to 500 μm.

was a mean clinical attachment level gain of 1.9 mm. The results of this study indicated that DFDBA has potential as a periodontal bone graft material and that a controlled clinical trial was needed.

## Clinical controlled studies

In a study by Mellonig (1984), DFDBA was procured and processed as previously described, and a total of 47 periodontal intraosseous defects were evaluated in 11 patients. Thirty-two lesions were implanted with DFDBA and 15 lesions were treated by open flap debridement alone. Each patient had at least one experimental and one control site. Matched-pair bilateral defects were selected if conditions permitted. Soft and hard tissue measurements for reduction in probing depth, clinical attachment gain, and bone fill were made before surgery and at the time of a 6- to 13-month surgical reentry.

There was 3.1 mm of probing depth reduction for sites treated by DFDBA and 2.86 mm for sites treated by open flap debridement. Both methods of treatment reduced pockets to an equal degree. The

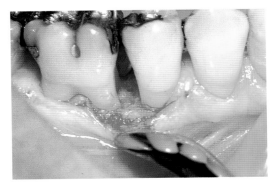

Fig 5-19c  Bone fill at the time of a 6-month postsurgical reentry. Figs 5-19a to c from Quintero et al 1982. Reprinted with permission.

significant difference was in the amount of gingival recession—0.2 for DFDBA and 1.3 for the control—and in clinical attachment gain—2.9 for DFDBA and 1.5 for the control. Hard tissue measurements yielded 2.6 mm (65%) bone fill in DFDBA sites and 1.3 mm (38%) in open flap debridement sites (Figs 5-20a to e). In addiiton, 78% of the sites treated by grafting showed greater than 50% or complete bone fill while only 40% of the control sites showed the same amount of bone fill.

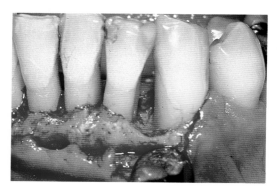

Fig 5-20a   Two-walled intraosseous defect on the mesial surface of the mandibular left canine.

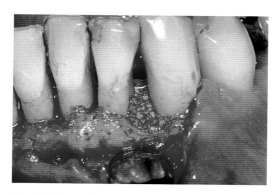

Fig 5-20b   Osseous defect implanted with decalcified freeze-dried bone allograft with a particle size of 250 to 1,000 μm.

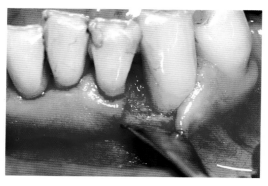

Fig 5-20c   Twelve-month postsurgery reentry showing complete osseous fill of the defect.

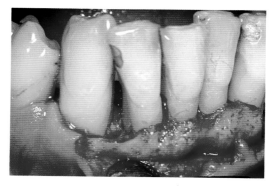

Fig 5-20d   Two-walled intraosseous control defect on the mesial surface of the mandibular right canine of the same patient.

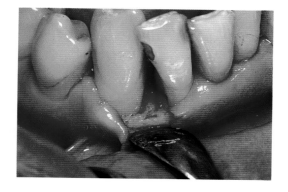

Fig 5-20e   Twelve-month reentry showing limited bone repair. Figs 5-20a to e from Mellonig 1984. Reprinted with permission.

## Histologic controlled studies

Although clinical controlled studies and case reports suggest efficacy for allogenic bone grafting, they do not indicate the type of attachment that occurs following a bone graft. The objective of the clinician who uses a bone graft is regeneration of the periodontium or new bone, cementum, and periodontal ligament around a root surface previously contaminated by bacterial plaque. Regeneration of a new attachment apparatus can only be demonstrated histologically.

Bowers et al (1989a) designed a three-part study in humans to answer the following questions:

1. Is regeneration of the attachment apparatus possible for periodontal intraosseous defects treated by open flap debridement?
2. Is regeneration of new bone, cementum, and periodontal ligament possible for defects treated by open flap debridement, crown removal, and submersion of the vital root beneath the mucosa?
3. Is regeneration enhanced if a bone graft is used for defects treated by open flap debridement, crown removal, and submersion of the vital root beneath the mucosa?
4. Is it possible to regenerate new bone, cementum, and periodontal ligament in defects treated by open flap debridement and DFDBA?

In part I of the study, the formation of new bone, cementum, and periodontal ligament was evaluated in open and closed environments (Bowers et al 1989a). The most apical level of calculus on the root surface was notched to indicate the pathologically exposed root. The mean distance between the base of the calculus and the base of the osseous defect was 3 mm. The average depth of all defects treated was 6 mm (Chadroff et al 1987). Teeth were either submerged or nonsubmerged. Teeth with submerged defects were treated by root planing, coronectomy, and submersion of vital teeth beneath the mucosa. Nonsubmerged teeth were treated by open flap debridement.

Biopsy specimens of experimental and control sites were obtained at 6 months after surgery from nine patients with 25 submerged and 22 nonsubmerged defects. Each patient acted as his or her own control. Test and control sites were evaluated histomorphometrically. Biopsy specimens were serially sectioned at 7 μm and every tenth section was stained. Linear measurements at magnification $\times$ 35 were made for the amount of regeneration from the base of the notch placed in calculus.

Results indicated that regeneration did not occur in any of the 22 nonsubmerged defects. Healing occurred by a long junctional epithelium (Fig 5-21). A new attachment apparatus did form in the submerged environment (0.75 mm), with 0.96 mm of new bone and 1.14 mm of new cementum (Fig 5-22).

These results indicated that periodontal regeneration is possible even if a bone graft is not used as long as epithelium can be excluded during healing. It now became important to determine the value of a bone graft in enhancing the formation of a new attachment apparatus.

In phase II of the study (Bowers et al 1989b), the healing of intraosseous defects with and without the addition of a DFDBA bone graft was evaluated in the submerged environment. The most apical level of calculus on the root surface served as a histologic reference point to measure regeneration on the root surfaces exposed to the oral environment. Grafted and nongrafted teeth both received root planing, coronectomy, and vital submergence beneath the oral mucosa. Biopsy speci-

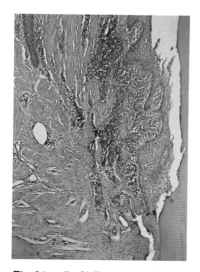 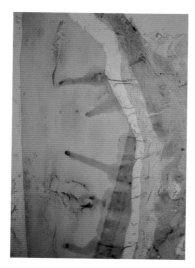

Fig 21 *(Left)* Representative section on nonsubmerged defect after open flap debridement. Note that location of the junctional epithelium is apical to the calculus notch. (Hematoxylin and eosin stain; original magnification × 25.)

Fig 5-22 *(Right)* Submerged defect showing the formation of new attachment apparatus from the calculus reference notch to the cut surface of the tooth. (Hematoxylin and eosin stain; original magnification × 25.)

mens from 30 grafted and 13 nongrafted defects were taken 6 months after surgery and were serially sectioned and evaluated histometrically for regeneration.

The results indicated that in the submerged environment significantly more new attachment apparatus formed in grafted than nongrafted sites. New bone and new cementum occurred more frequently in grafted than in nongrafted defects (Figs 5-23 and 5-24). The periodontal ligament was oriented parallel, perpendicularly, or both in the same defect. No extensive root resorption, ankylosis, or pulp death was observed in grafted or nongrafted sites. This study clearly indicated that a graft of cortical DFDBA has an inductive effect on the formation of new bone, and that such a bone graft could stimulate connective tissue attachment to the root surface.

Part III of this study (Bowers et al 1989c) answered the following question. After open flap debridement of intraosseous defects and root planing of pathologically exposed root surfaces in a nonsubmerged environment, will DFDBA enhance formation of new bone, cementum, and periodontal ligament? A notch in calculus on the root surface served as a histologic reference point to delineate that portion of the root surface exposed to the oral environment. Data from 12 patients with 32 grafted and 25 nongrafted sites were evaluated. Biopsy specimens were obtained 6 months postsurgery and analyzed histometrically for regeneration of a new attachment apparatus.

A mean new attachment apparatus was formed, 1.21 mm from the calculus notch in DFDBA grafted sites and 0.00 mm from

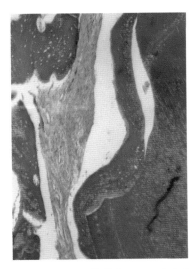 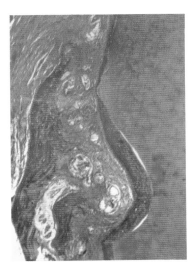

Fig 5-23   *(Left)* Submerged defect implanted with decalcified freeze-dried bone allograft showing formation of a new bone, cementum, and periodontal ligament from the calculus reference notch. (Trichrome stain; original magnification × 25.)

Fig 5-24   *(Right)* Submerged nongrafted defect showing formation of a new attachment apparatus from the calculus reference notch. (Trichrome stain; original magnification × 25.)

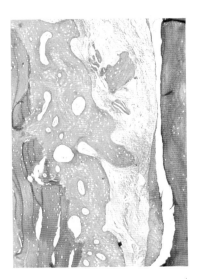 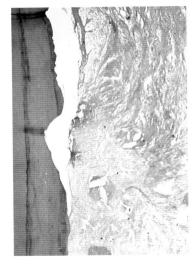

Fig 5-25   *(Left)* Nonsubmerged grafted defect showing formation of new bone, cementum, and periodontal ligament from the calculus reference notch. (Hematoxylin and eosin stain; original magnification × 25.)

Fig 5-26   *(Right)* Nonsubmerged nongrafted defect showing healing by a long junctional epithelium. (Hematoxylin and eosin stain; original magnification × 25.)

93

the notch in defects treated by open flap debridement alone. There was more new cementum (1.24 mm) and more new bone (1.75 mm) in grafted sites than in nongrafted sites (0.00 mm for both new bone and cementum) (Figs 5-25 and 5-26).

This series of 147 human biopsy specimens conclusively demonstrated that *(1)* regeneration of the periodontium can occur on pathologically exposed roots; *(2)* a bone graft can induce more regeneration even under conditions normally conducive to this phenomenon; and *(3)* a bone graft will enhance the amount and frequency of regeneration in the both submerged and nonsubmerged environments.

# Comparison of bone allografts and bone substitutes

The next series of studies set out to answer the following questions. How do FDBA and DFDBA compare to a synthetic bone graft material when used to treat periodontal bone defects? How do FDBA and DFDBA compare to each other?

Granular porous hydroxyapatite is considered a unique alloplast or bone substitute in that it is formed by the hydrothermal chemical conversion of sea coral from biogenic carbonate to hydroxyapatite (White and Shore 1986). This gives it an inorganic content similar to that of bone. A microstructure similar to that of bone (pore size of 190 to 230 µm) facilitates vascular ingrowth and subsequent new bone formation (Chiroff et al 1975). Studies of porous hydroxyapatite indicate that a bone repair of 3.5 mm is obtainable in grafted sites while only 0.7 mm is obtainable in nongrafted defects (Kenney et al 1985). In the treatment of furcation lesions, significant improvement in attachment level and fill of bone defects compared with that found in control defects has also been reported

(Kenney et al 1988). Therefore, this alloplast would appear to be a likely substitute for FDBA or DFDBA.

In a study by Barnett et al (1989), 19 pairs of intraosseous defects were grafted in seven patients. One defect of each pair was implanted with FDBA, the other with porous particulate hydroxyapatite (PHA). Paired defects were treated similarly in all aspects. Measurements were made for probing depth, clinical attachment level, and osseous changes. All sites were reentered 6 to 11 months postsurgery and all measurements were repeated.

Results showed an average bone fill of 2.1 mm (66%) for FDBA and 1.3 mm (42%) for PHA (Figs 5-27a to c). Also found was a mean clinical attachment gain of 2.2 mm for FDBA and 1.3 mm for PHA, and an average reduction in probing depth of 3.0 mm for FDBA and 1.4 mm for PHA. This data suggested that FDBA may have better reparative potential than PHA for the treatment of periodontal osseous defects.

The second phase of this study compared DFDBA to PHA (Bowen et al 1989). Six patients with advanced periodontitis and at least two comparable osseous lesions participated. Each subject received initial therapy consisting of oral hygiene instruction, scaling, root planing, and occlusal adjustment as indicated. Baseline measurements were made during the posthygiene phase of therapy and consisted of probing depth, clinical attachment levels, and gingival recession. Alveolar crest height and depth of osseous lesion were obtained at the time of surgery. All measurements were made from a fixed reference point and repeated at the time of a 6-month reentry surgery. Thirty-four osseous defects (17 pairs) were implanted with either DFDBA or PHA. Each patient acted as his or her own control. There were no significant differences in any of the soft tissue measurements when DFDBA and PHA were compared. However, both treat-

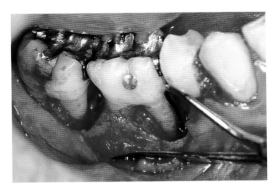

Fig 5-27a   Surgical exposure of implant sites (mesial surface of the mandibular right first and second molars) prior to implantation of graft materials.

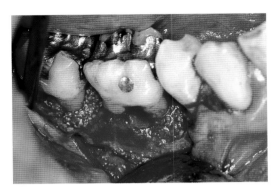

Fig 5-27b   Freeze-dried bone allograft in the mesial surface of the first molar and porous particulate hydroxyapatite in the mesial surface of the second molar.

ment modalities reduced probing depth and demonstrated a gain in clinical attachment levels. There was 2.2 mm (61%) bone fill with DFDBA and 2.1 mm (53%) bone repair with PHA. These values were likewise not clinically significant (Figs 5-28a and b and 5-29a and b).

The third phase of this investigation compared FDBA and DFDBA (Rummelhart et al 1989). Twenty-two bone defects (11 intrapatient pairs) in nine patients were grafted with either FDBA or DFDBA. Evaluations were based on presurgical and postsurgical soft tissue measurements and hard tissue measurements at surgery and a 6-month reentry.

An average bone fill of 1.7 mm (59%) occurred with DFDBA and 2.4 mm (66%) with FDBA. Soft tissue measurements demonstrated a probing depth reduction of 2.4 mm and a clinical attachment gain of 1.7 mm for DFDBA; for FDBA the measurements were 2.3 mm probing depth reduction and 2.0 mm clinical attachment gain. These findings reveal no significant differences between the two materials in primarily one-walled osseous defects.

The results of these studies indicated that there may be limited differences

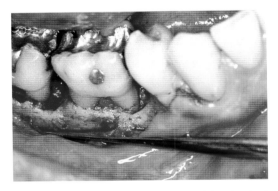

Fig 5-27c   Surgical exposure of implanted sites at 6 months postsurgery.

between DFDBA, FDBA, and PHA in probing depth reduction, clinical attachment gain, and bone fill. However, histologically there are major differences. Evidence exists that grafts of DFDBA may heal by regenerating the periodontium.

Human histology demonstrates that connective tissue tends to encapsulate hydroxyapatite grafts with minimal or no bone formation (Froum et al 1982). Bone formation has occurred alongside and within the graft particles (Kenney et al

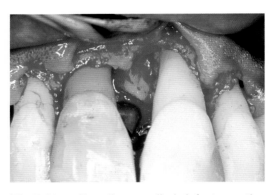

Fig 5-28a   Two three-walled defects on the mesial surface of the left maxillary central incisor prior to grafting with decalcified freeze-dried bone allograft.

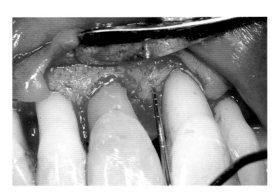

Fig 5-28b   At 6-month reentry, a 3-mm bone fill was recorded.

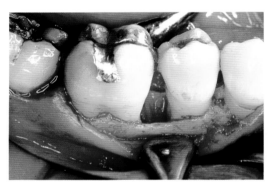

Fig 5-29a   Two-walled crater on the mesial surface of the mandibular first molar prior to implantation with particulate porous hydroxyapatite.

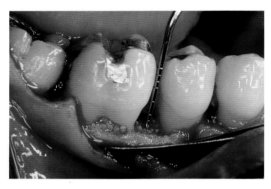

Fig 5-29b   At 6-month reentry, bone repair is complete but particles of hydroxyapatite firmly encased in hard tissue can be noted.

1986), but there is no definitive evidence that hydroxyapatite regenerates the periodontium (Carranza et al 1987).

The choice between graft materials may then be dependent on other factors, such as the possibility for disease transfer following a bone allograft. This possibility is highly unlikely if a tissue bank uses medical and social screening, antibody testing, direct antigen tests, serologic tests, bacter- ial culturing, autopsy, and follow-up study of grafts from the same donor. If these exclusionary techniques are used, the chances of transmitting a disease are approximately 1 in 1.67 million (Buck et al 1989). Processing the allograft reduces the risk to 1 in 8 million (Buck et al 1990; Quinnan et al 1986; Resnick et al 1986). A recent study (Mellonig et al 1992) demonstrated that treatment of a cortical bone allograft with a virucidal agent and demineralization will inactivate the AIDS virus even if present.

# Decalcified freeze-dried bone allografts and guided tissue regeneration

Wound healing studies in animals suggest that if a periodontal lesion is repopulated by cells from either the gingival epithelium, gingival connective tissue, or alveolar bone, a long junctional epithelium, root resorption, or ankylosis will result (Karring et al 1980, 1984; Nyman et al 1980). A physical barrier of membrane composed of expanded polytetrafluoroethylene (ePTFE) placed between the mucogingival flap and the root surface will retard apical migration of epithelium, prevent gingival connective tissue from contacting the root surface, and promote migration of cells from the periodontal ligament (Gottlow et al 1986). This wound healing principle is known as guided tissue regeneration (GTR).

Clinical trials indicate that intraosseous and furcation lesions can be corrected with this technique (Becker et al 1988; Pontoriero et al 1988). The lesions are filled with tissue with the consistency of rubber and are resistant to penetration of a periodontal probe. Human histologic observations suggest that GTR favors a new connective attachment with little or no bone formation.

Recent studies indicate that periodontal ligament cells migrate a short distance, and at the same rate, with or without the placement of a physical barrier (Aukhil et al 1988). Therefore, the critical role of the periodontal membrane may be that of space creation to allow migrating cells sufficient time to undergo amplifying cell division and populate the root surface (Aukhil et al 1988). Furthermore, cells from bone may play a major role in GTR. Cells from the endosteal spaces of alveolar bone can synthesize cementumlike tissue and may migrate from bone into the periodontal ligament. The addition of a bone graft to the GTR technique may then serve to hold the space, retain the blood clot, provide a matrix over which cells can migrate, and induce the differentiation of cells into osteoblasts.

Andereg et al (1991) investigated the potential of DFDBA combined with an ePTFE membrane to cause bone fill as compared to the membrane alone. Fifteen pairs of class II furcation lesions (30 defects) in 15 patients made up the study group. Soft and hard tissue measurements of probing depth reduction, recession, attachment level gain, and osseous defect fill of bone served as clinical parameters for comparison. The ePTFE membranes were removed 4 to 6 weeks postinsertion.

Six months posttreatment, each site was surgically reentered and measurements were repeated. There was 0.9 mm of recession, 3.1 mm of clinical attachment gain, and 3.1 mm of probing depth reduction for sites treated by both DFDBA and the ePTFE. Sites treated with the membrane alone showed 0.8 mm of recession, 1.4 mm of attachment gain, and 2.2 mm of probing depth reduction. Hard tissue measurements demonstrated 3.5 mm of vertical bone fill and 2.4 mm of horizontal fill. Control defects showed 1.7 mm of vertical and 1.0 mm of horizontal bone fill (Figs 5-30a to c and 5-31a to c). These differences were statistically significant in favor of using the combined DFDBA plus ePTFE technique.

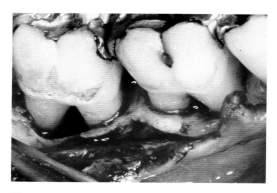

Fig 5-30a Class II furcation invasion defects on the facial surface of both the mandibular first and second molars.

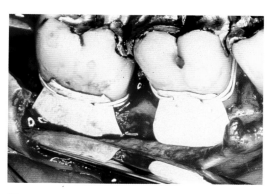

Fig 5-30b Furcation on the second molar was treated with the expanded-polytetrafluoroethylene membrane alone, whereas the first molar was treated with a decalcified freeze-dried bone allograft. Contralateral defects were treated in an opposite manner.

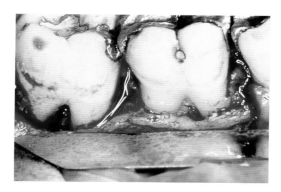

Fig 5-30c Reentry of the furcation defects to bone at 6 months demonstrated bone fill of the defect treated by membrane and bone graft. Note the limited bone fill of the defect treated by the membrane alone.

## Future directions

Little difference exists in the clinical results achieved with FDBA and DFDBA (Rummelhart et al 1989). Animal studies suggest that DFDBA should have greater osteogenic potential (Mellonig et al 1981). A possible reason for the discrepancy between animal and human data may be that there is not enough bone-inductive protein, such as BMP, in a human periodontal bone graft to exert any appreciable effect on bone growth. The minimum effective dose of BMP is approximately 2 μg/40 mg (wet weight) of explant (Sato and Urist 1983). The optimum dose is about 10 μg. Therefore, the DFDBA bone graft may have to be augmented with inductive proteins to realize the potential demonstrated in the animal model.

Such a bone-inductive protein may be osteogenin. Osteogenin is a member of the bone morphogenetic family of proteins and has been isolated from the extracellular bone matrix of humans (Luyten et al 1989; Sampath and Reddi 1987). It has homology with BMP-3 expressed from recombinant BMP (Wozney et al 1988).

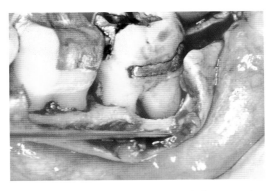

Fig 5-31a   Class II furcation defect on the facial surface of the mandibular left first molar.

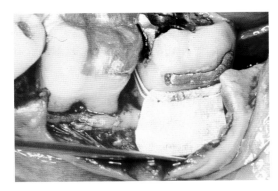

Fig 5-31b   Defect treated by expanded-polytetrafluoroethylene membrane and a decalcified freeze-dried bone allograft.

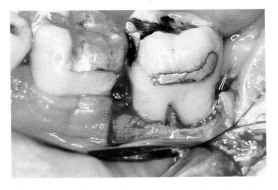

Fig 5-31c   Six-month surgical reentry showing bone fill of the furcation lesion.

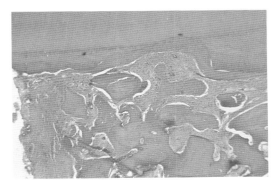

Fig 5-32   Representative section of submerged defect treated with decalcified freeze-dried bone allograft plus the bone-inductive protein, osteogenin. Note complete reformation of attachment apparatus coronal to the notch placed in calculus. (Hematoxylin and eosin stain; original magnification × 25.)

Osteogenin in association with a bone-derived matrix will rapidly initiate the cascade of bone formation (Reddi et al 1987; Vukicevic et al 1989). The potential application of such a growth factor in periodontics appears to be promising.

Bowers et al (1991) compared DFDBA with DFDBA plus osteogenin in 36 submerged and 50 nonsubmerged defects in 14 patients. The most apical level of calculus on the root served as the histologic ref-

erence point to measure regeneration. They found that the combination of osteogenin plus DFDBA significantly enhanced regeneration of a new attachment apparatus (1.92 mm) compared to DFDBA alone (1.31 mm) in the submerged environment (Fig 5-32). Osteogenin plus DFDBA also enhanced regeneration in a nonsubmerged environment (2.33 mm) compared to DFDBA alone (1.72 mm), but these differences were not statistically significant. It is clear that such combinations of bone and inductive proteins or combinations of other polypeptides, such as platelet-derived and insulinlike growth factors, will have major importance in future regenerative attempts (Lynch et al 1989).

# References

Andereg CR, Marten SJ, Gray JL, Mellonig JT, Gher ME. Clinical evaluation of the use of decalcified freeze-dried bone allograft with guided tissue regeneration in the treatment of molar furcation invasions. *J Periodontol* 1991;62:264–268.

Aukhil I, Iglhaut J. Periodontal ligament cell kinetics following experimental regenerative procedures. *J Clin Periodont* 1988;15:374–382.

Barnett J, Mellonig J, Towle H, Gray J. Comparison of freeze-dried bone allograft and porous hydroxyapatite in human periodontal defects. *J Periodontol* 1989;60:231–237.

Becker W, Becker B, Berg C, Prichard J, Caffesse R, Rosenberg E. New attachment after treatment with root isolation procedures: report for treated class III and class II furcations and vertical osseous defects. *Int J Periodont Rest Dent* 1988;8(3):9–24.

Bhaskar SN, Cutright DE, Knapp MJ, Beasley JD, Perez B, Driskell TD. Tissue reaction to intrabony ceramic implants. *Oral Surg Oral Med Oral Pathol* 1971;31:282–289.

Bowen J, Mellonig J, Gray J, Towle H. Comparison of decalcified freeze-dried bone allograft and porous particulate hydroxyapatite in human periodontal osseous defects *J Periodontol* 1989;60:647–654.

Bowers G, Chadroff B, Carnevale R, et al. Histologic evaluation of new human attachment apparatus formation in humans, Part I. *J Periodontol* 1989a; 60:664–674.

Bowers G, Chadroff B, Carnevale R, et al. Histologic evaluation of new human attachment apparatus in humans, Part II. *J Periodontol* 1989b;60:675–682.

Bowers G, Chadroff B, Carnevale R, et al. Histologic evaluation of new human attachment apparatus in humans, Part III. *J Periodontol* 1989c;60:683–693.

Bowers G, Felton F, Middleton C, et al. Histologic comparison of regeneration in human intrabony defects when osteogenin is combined with demineralized freeze-dried bone allograft and with purified bovine collagen. *J Periodontol* 1991; 62:690–702.

Buck B, Malinin T, Brown M. Bone transplantation and human immunodeficiency virus; an estimate of risk-acquired immunodeficiency syndrome (AIDS). *Clin Orthop* 1989;240:129–134.

Buck B, Resnick B, Shah S, Malinin T. Human immunodeficiency virus cultured from bone. Implications for transplantation. *Clin Orthop* 1990;251:249–253.

Carranza R, Kenney E, Lekovic V, Talamante E, Valencia J, Dimitrijevic B. Histologic study of healing of human periodontal defects after placement of porous hydroxyapatite implants. *J Periodontol* 1987;58:682–688.

Caton J, Kowalski CJ. Primate model for testing periodontal treatment procedures II. Production of contralaterally similar lesions. *J Periodontol* 1976;47:71–77.

Chadroff B, Bowers G, Richardson AC. The apical location of calculus within the intrabony defect. *J Dent Res* 1987;60 (special issue A):338.

Chiroff R, White D, Weber J, Roy D. The ingrowth of replamineform implants. *J Biomed Mater Res* 1975;6:29.

Diem CR, Bowers GM, Moffitt WC. Bone blending: a technique for bone implantation. *J Periodontol* 1972;43:295–297.

Elves MW. An evaluation of the use of strontium 85 for the assessment of experimental bone grafts. *Acta Orthop Scand* 1974;45:641–646.

Frielaender GE, Strong DM, Sell KW. Studies on the antigenicity of bone. II. Donor-specific anti-HLA antibodies in human recipients of freeze-dried allografts. *J Bone Joint Surg* 1984;66-A:107–111.

Froum SJ, Thaler R, Scopp IW, Stahl SS. Osseous autografts. Part I: Clinical responses to bone blend or hip marrow grafts. *J Periodontol* 1975; 46:516–521.

Froum SJ, Ortiz M, Witkins RT, Thaler R, Scopp IW, Stahl SS. Osseous autografts. III. Comparison of osseous coagulum-bone blend implants with open curettage. *J Periodontol* 1976;47:287–294.

Froum S, Kushner L, Scopp I, Stahl S. Human clinical and histologic responses to Durapatite implants in intraosseous lesions. Case reports. *J Periodontol* 1982;53:719–725.

Goldberg VM, Stevenson S. Natural history of autografts and allografts. *Clin Orthop* 1987;225:7–16.

Gottlow J, Nyman S, Lindhe J, Karring T, Winnestrom J. New attachment formation in the human periodontium by guided tissue regeneration. *J Clin Periodontol* 1986;13:604–616.

Harakas N. Demineralized bone-matrix-induced osteogenesis. *Clin Orthop* 1984;188:239–251.

Hulbert SF, Young FA, Mathews RS, Klawitter JJ, Talbert CD, Stelling FJ. Potential of ceramic materials as permanently implantable skeletal prosthesis. *J Biomed Mater Res* 1970;4:433–456.

Karring T, Nyman S, Lindhe J. Healing following implantation of periodontitis affected roots into bone tissue. *J Clin Periodontol* 1980;7:96–105.

Karring T, Nyman S, Lindhe J, Sirirat M. Potentials for root resorption during periodontal wound healing. *J Clin Periodontol* 1984;11:41–52.

Kenney EB, Lekovic V, Han T, Carranza F, Dimitrijevic B. The use of a porous hydroxyapatite implant in periodontal defects. I. Clinical results after six months. *J Periodontol* 1985;56:82–88.

Kenney E, Lekovic V, Ferrira C, Han T, Dimitrijevic B, Carranza F. Bone formation within porous hydroxyapatite implants in human periodontal defects. *J Periodontol* 1986;57:76–83.

Kenney EB, Lekovic V, Elbaz J, Kovacvic K, Carranza F, Takei H. The use of a porous hydroxyapatite implant in periodontal defects. II. Treatment of class II furcation lesions in lower molars. *J Periodontol* 1988;59:67–72.

Luyten FP, Cunningham NS, Na S, et al. Purification and partial amino sequence of osteogenin, a protein initiating bone differentiation. *J Biol Chem* 1989;264:13377–13380.

Lynch SE, Williams RC, Polson AM, et al. A combination of platelet-derived and insulin-like growth factors enhances periodontal regeneration. *J Clin Periodontol* 1989;16:545–548.

Mellonig J, Bowers G, Bright R, Lawrence J. Clinical evaluation of freeze-dried bone allograft in periodontal osseous defects. *J Periodontol* 1976;47:125–129.

Mellonig JT, Bowers GM, Baily RC, Levy RA. New bone formation with autograft-allograft composites. *J Dent Res* 1980;59 (special issue A):872.

Mellonig JT. Histological evaluation of freeze-dried bone allograft in periodontal osseous defects of baboons. *J Dent Res* 1981;61 (special issue A):311.

Mellonig J, Bowers G, Baily R. Comparison of bone graft materials. I. New bone formation with autografts and allografts determined by strontium 85. *J Periodontol* 1981a;52:291–296.

Mellonig J, Bowers G, Cotton W. Comparison of bone graft materials. Part II. New bone formation with autografts and allografts: A histological evaluation. *J Periodontol* 1981b;52:297–302.

Mellonig JT, Bowers GM, Branham G. Histologic evaluation of autograft-allograft composites. *J Dent Res* 1982;61 (special issue A):1442.

Mellonig JT, Bowers GM, Levy RA, Branham G. Radionuclide and histological evaluation of marrow-allograft composites. *J Dent Res* 1983; 62 (special issue A):1208.

Mellonig JT, Levy RA. Effect of different particle sizes of freeze-dried bone allograft on the rate of bone growth. *J Dent Res* 1984;63 (special issue A):461.

Mellonig JT. Decalcified freeze-dried bone allograft as an implant material in human periodontal defects. *Int J Periodont Rest Dent* 1984;4(6):41–55.

Mellonig JT, Prewitt AM, Moyer MP. HIV inactivation in a bone allograft. *J Periodontol* 1992;63:979–983.

Nyman S, Karring T, Lindhe J, Planten S. Healing following implantation of periodontitis affected roots into gingival connective tissue. *J Clin Periodontol* 1980;7:394–401.

Pontoriero R, Lindhe J, Nyman S, Karring T, Rosenberg E, Sanavi R. Guided tissue regeneration in degree II furcation involved mandibular molars. *J Clin Periodontol* 1988;15:247–254.

Quattlebaum J, Mellonig J, Hansel N. Antigenicity of freeze-dried cortical bone allograft in human periodontal osseous defects. *J Periodontol* 1988; 59:394–397.

Quinnan G, Wells J, Wittek M. Inactivation of human T-cell lymphotropic virus, Type III by heat chemicals and irradiation. *Transfusion* 1986;26: 481–483.

Quintero G, Mellonig J, Gambill V. A six month clinical evaluation of decalcified freeze-dried bone allograft in human periodontal defects. *J Periodontol* 1982;53:726–730.

Reddi AH, Wientroub S, Muthukmuaran N. Biologic principles of bone induction. *Orthop Clin North Am* 1987;18:207–212.

Resnick L, Veren K, Salahuddin, Tondeau S, Markham P. Stability and inactivation of HTLV-III/LAV under clinical and laboratory environments. *JAMA* 1986;255:1987–1991.

Robinson RE. Osseous coagulum for bone induction. *J Periodontol* 1969;40:503–510.

Rummelhart J, Mellonig J, Gray T, Gray J. Comparison of freeze-dried bone allograft in human periodontal osseous defects. *J Periodontol* 1989;60:655–663.

Sampath T, Reddi A. Homology of bone inductive proteins from human, monkey, bovine, and rat extracellular matrix. *Proc Natl Acad Sci USA* 1983;80:6591–6595.

Sanders J, Sepe W, Bowers G, et al. Clinical evaluation of freeze-dried bone allograft in periodontal osseous defects. III. Composite freeze-dried bone allografts with and without autogenous bone grafts. *J Periodontol* 1983;54:1–11.

Sato K, Urist MR. Bone morphogenetic protein induced cartilage development in tissue culture. *Clin Orthop* 1984;183:180–187.

Schallhorn RG. Present status of osseous grafting procedures. *J Periodontol* 1977;48:570–576.

Sepe W, Bowers G, Lawrence J, Friedlaender G, Kock R. Clinical evaluation of freeze-dried bone allografts in periodontal osseous defects. *J Periodontol* 1978;49:9–14.

Shapoff C, Bowers GM, Levy B, Mellonig J, Yukna R. The effect of particle size on the osteogenic activity of composite grafts of allogenic freeze-dried bone allograft and autogenous marrow. *J Periodontol* 1980;51:625–630.

Topazian RG, Hammer WB, Boucher LJ, Hubert SF. Use of alloplasts for ridge augmentation. *J Oral Surg* 1971;29:792–798.

Turner D, Mellonig JT. Antigenicity of freeze-dried bone allograft in periodontal osseous defects. *J Periodont Res* 1981;16:89–99.

Urist MR. Bone formation by autoinduction. *Science* 1965;150:893–899.

Urist MR, Silverman BF, Burning K, Dubuc FL, Rosenberg JM. The bone induction principle. *Clin Orthop* 1967;53:243–264.

Urist MR, Dowell TA, Hay PH, Strates BS. Inductive substrates for bone formation. *Clin Orthop* 1968;59:59–96.

Urist MR, Dowell TA. Inductive substratum for osteogenesis in pellets of particulate bone matrix. *Clin Orthop* 1968;61:61–78.

Urist MR, Jurist J, Ducuc T, Strates B. Quantitation of new bone formation in intramuscular implants of bone matrix in rabbits. *Clin Orthop* 1970;68:279–293.

Urist MR, Strates B. Bone formation in implants of partially and wholly demineralized bone matrix. *Clin Orthop* 1970;71:271–278.

Urist MR, Strates B. Bone morphogenetic protein. *J Dent Res* 1971;50:1392–1406.

Urist MR, Mikulski A, Boyd SD. A chemosterilized antigen-extracted autodigested alloimplant for bone banks. *Arch Surg* 1975;110:416–428.

Urist MR, Sato K, Brownell A, et al. Human bone morphogenetic protein (hBMP). *Proc Soc Exp Biol Med* 1983;173:194–199.

Vukicevic V, Rosen V, Celeste AJ, et al. Stimulation of the expression of osteogenic and chrondrogenic phenotypes in vitro by osteogenin. *Proc Natl Acad Sci USA* 1988;86:8793–8797.

White E, Shore EC. Biomaterial aspects of Interpore 200 porous hydroxyapatite. *Dent Clin North Am* 1989;30:49–59.

Wozney J, Rosen V, Celeste A, et al. Novel regulators of bone formation: molecular clones and activities. *Science* 1988;242:1528–1534.

Chapter 6

# Synthetic Grafts and Regeneration

Raymond A. Yukna

The reconstruction or restoration of osseous defects caused by inflammatory periodontal disease is a continuing challenge in periodontal therapy. Although many attempts have been made to regenerate alveolar bone support and the attachment apparatus, predictable success has proved elusive. Historically, autogenous and/or allogenic graft materials have been used with moderate success (Dragoo and Sullivan 1973; Froum et al 1975; Hiatt and Schallhorn 1973; Mellonig 1984; Schallhorn et al 1970; Schallhorn 1977; Sepe et al 1978). It is often difficult to procure sufficient autogenous bone and there is some concern about the possibility (albeit remote) of disease transfer with freeze-dried bone allografts.

Osseous grafts are the only type for which ample histologic evidence is available of periodontal reconstruction in humans, including new cementum, alveolar bone, and a functional periodontal ligament (Bowers et al 1989; Nabers et al 1972; Ross and Cohen 1968). Despite the success demonstrated with transplants of osseous material, however, the use of such grafts is frequently either impractical or impossible.

The ideal graft material remains to be found. Such a material would induce osteogenesis and cementogenesis that would result in regeneration of a new periodontal attachment complex at a more coronal level. It would be completely biocompatible and would not be carcinogenic, toxic, antigenic, or effect round-cell infiltration responses. It would also be easily obtainable, relatively inexpensive, and would not cause the patient or the surgeon unnecessary inconvenience.

## Development of synthetic graft materials

An inorganic synthetic material would seem to fulfill the criteria for an "ideal" graft material. Several alloplastic implant materials have been used in an attempt to improve clinical conditions and regenerate bone in periodontal infrabony defects (Table 6-1). The most successful of these materials have been ceramics of either the bioresorbable or nonresorbable type.

103

Table 6-1    Alloplastic graft materials

> Plaster of Paris
> Polymers
> Calcium carbonates
> Ceramics
>> Resorbable—
>>> Tricalcium phosphate
>>> Resorbable hydroxyapatite
>> Nonresorbable—
>>> Dense hydroxyapatite
>>> Porous hydroxyapatite
>>> Bioglass

Early studies using calcium phosphate materials focused on the principle that local release of calcium ions would stimulate bone formation at the site. These early studies with soluble calcium powders yielded equivocal results and led to further studies with tricalcium phosphate (TCP) and modified forms of hydroxyapatite (HA), the latter usually having a β-whitlockite crystal structure (Jarcho 1981).

Clinical results with synthetic graft materials are essentially similar to results obtained with autogenous or allogenic materials, both in direct comparative studies and in cross-sectional comparisons of similar evaluations and studies. The choice of material then becomes based more on availability, cost, morbidity, and ease of handling than on clinical superiority.

The available alloplastic materials can be classified generally as resorbable or nonresorbable. In general terms, plaster of Paris, calcium carbonate, tricalcium phosphate, and "resorbable" hydroxyapatite resorb totally or partially in oral and periodontal surgery sites, whereas the polymers and dense hydroxyapatites do not. There is some controversy as to which of these biologic results is preferable in dental usage, and selection of one type or another may depend on the actual clinical application. All of the commercially available allo-plastics listed in Table 6-1, except plaster of Paris, have a particle size between 300 to 500 μm in diameter. This particle size is thought to be optimum for periodontal usage (Zaner and Yukna 1984).

Animal and human wound healing studies have uniformly demonstrated the biocompatibility of the listed alloplastic materials. A lack of local or systemic toxicity, a lack of inflammatory or foreign body response, and the ability to become directly bonded to bone are all positive attributes of these materials (Boetto and Freeman 1984; Bowers et al 1989; Frank et al 1987; Froum et al 1982; Jarcho 1981; Meffert et al 1986; Sapkos 1986).

# Rationale for use of synthetic grafts in periodontics

The decision to use alloplastic grafting materials during surgical periodontal treatment is made on the same basis as the decision to graft. Those practitioners who have advanced training or extensive experience in periodontal surgical techniques and who entertain a reconstructive philosophy are likely users of synthetic or other bone grafting materials.

Periodontal bony defects are treated because they complicate the definitive elimination of active pocket defects, compromise the support of the tooth and the tooth's ability to withstand functional stresses, and complicate maintenance of an arrested pocket defect. The ideal result is correction of bony defects by regeneration of lost supporting bone and periodontal ligament (Figs 6-1a to d).

At present, bone grafting is the only modality of therapy for which there is histologic evidence, in humans, of regeneration of new attachment composed of new bone, new cementum, and new periodontal ligament coronal to the base of a previous osseous defect. This does not imply that all bone grafts are uniformly successful,

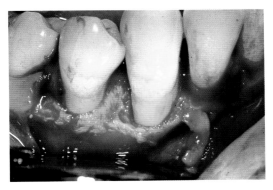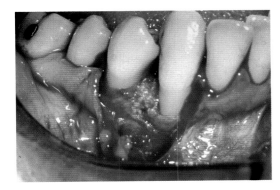

Figs 6-1a to 1d   Clinical example of results with hydroxyapatite bone replacement graft material on distofacial portion of mandibular right canine of a 36-year-old woman.

Fig 6-1a   *(Left)* Surgical exposure of combination 1-2-3 wall defect measuring 4 mm from alveolar crest to base of defect.

Fig 6-1b   *(Right)* Appearance of repaired defect at 6-month reentry. Note the granular appearance of the filled area with evidence of ceramic granules near the surface.

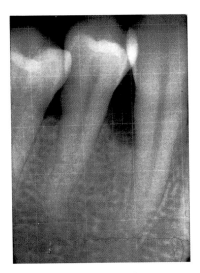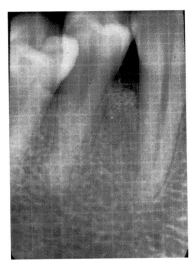

Fig 6-1c   Presurgical radiograph.

Fig 6-1d   Six-month postoperative radiograph. Note the volume of the radiodense ceramic evidence in the area of the original defect.

routinely predictable, or will heal with restoration of the entire attachment complex. Partial repair often occurs with adherence of a long junctional epithelium to the root surface and/or adhesion of connective tissue fibers oriented parallel to the root. Nevertheless, regeneration of a complete new attachment occurs frequently enough with bone grafts to warrant their use in selective cases. Guided tissue regeneration techniques, on the other hand, do not appear to induce the formation of periodontal supporting bone (Becker et al 1988; Gottlow et al 1986).

Furthermore, there is evidence that supracrestal bone regeneration is possible when certain bone grafting materials are used. This has not been observed with other forms of regenerative periodontal therapy that attempt to eliminate bony defects without an osseous graft material (Dragoo and Sullivan 1973; Mellonig 1982; Sapkos 1986).

Following are indications for use of bone grafts as part of surgical periodontal pocket therapy (Mellonig 1982):

1. Deep infrabony defects associated with chronic inflammatory periodontal disease may be treated with bone grafts. While narrow three-walled defects may respond equally well to grafting or debridement (flap curettage) alone, the response of wide three-walled, two-walled, one-walled, and combination defects is enhanced by the addition of bone grafts.
2. Increased bone support for a tooth may be achieved with bone grafts. Such procedures may restore sufficient functional stability to make the tooth an acceptable abutment for restorative dentistry and preserve arch integrity.
3. Lesions associated with localized juvenile periodontitis have consistently and successfully been treated with bone grafts. Use of bone grafts in patients with this condition has eliminated the wholesale extraction of involved teeth and has often regenerated almost the entire amount of previously lost bone.
4. Maintenance of, or esthetic transformation of, gingival margin height may be an important goal of bone grafting. If periodontal pockets associated with shallow bone defects are treated by osseous resection and apically positioned flaps, the resultant longer clinical crowns may be esthetically unacceptable. Reconstruction of these defects with bone grafts and the subsequent retention of the gingival margin close to the cementoenamel junction may preserve esthetics.

Bone grafts are indicated for those patients who have the time for a rigorous treatment regimen and postsurgical maintenance program. The use of bone grafts is also dictated by patient acceptance, economic factors, availability of graft material, past experience with bone grafting procedures, and patient selection. The practitioner's lack of clinical experience often leads to discouraging results. Moreover, bone grafts are only indicated when the patient has met the practitioner's criteria for selection.

## Patient selection

Patient selection is particularly important in the use and success of bone grafts. The patient must be highly motivated and demonstrate his or her ability to effectively remove bacterial plaque from every surface of every tooth on a daily basis. Baseline records and a plaque index are essential in determining the patient's progress. The patient's attitude toward therapy must be positive. Treatment should be accepted as a worthwhile investment of time and effort in himself or herself. The patient's gingival tissue response to initial preparation should be indicative of some resolution of inflammation. Likewise, the patient's age, health, emotional status, social habits (such as smoking), and tolerance for lengthy dental appointments are important considerations. These criteria will limit the number of patients who are good candidates for this type of therapy. Unless these factors are favorable, the clinician invites failure, and bone grafts may be contraindicated.

# Bone graft technique

The general surgical technique used in periodontal bone grafting uses many of the same basic, tedious, painstaking procedures that are also used for other forms of periodontal surgery. While not a guarantee of success, the following steps in the procedure provide a road map that leads toward success a majority of the time.

**1. Removal of all etiologic factors.** Local and systemic factors must be under control for bone grafts to be successful. This control would optimally have been accomplished presurgically.

**2. Stabilization of teeth, if necessary.** Generally, provisional or permanent stabilization of teeth undergoing bone grafts is not necessary. Teeth with slight to moderate mobility appear to heal just as well whether or not they are splinted. However, extremely mobile teeth that are being treated in an attempt to retain them may benefit from provisional stabilization for at least 6 months postsurgically. At the very least, this stabilization allows proper control of the occlusion and the performance of therapeutic measures such as root planing.

**3. Creation of a flap design with a plan for closure.** Internally beveled scalloped incisions with full gingival retention are necessary to be able to completely close the site at the completion of surgery. Full-thickness flaps, reflected beyond the mucogingival junction, are recommended. Vertical releasing incisions should be used

as necessary to allow proper access to the defects (Fig 6-2a).

**4. Degranulation of defect and flap.** All granulomatous soft tissues should be removed from the bony walls of the defect and the associated tooth surfaces (Fig 6-2b). Also, the inner aspect of the flap should be checked for tissue tags and epithelial remnants.

**5. Preparation of the root.** It is essential that all calculus, bacterial plaque, other soft debris and altered cementum be removed from the involved root surfaces. Ultrasonic and hand instruments as well as burs are useful for this purpose. This aspect of therapy is the most tedious, difficult, and time-consuming of the entire procedure (Fig 6-2b). It is also the most essential aspect. The use of chemicals such as citric acid or tetracycline paste may be an aid in root detoxification and in making the root surface more biologically acceptable for healing (see chapter 4).

**6. Promotion of a bleeding bony surface.** This is generally already accomplished by proper defect debridement. However, if the defect walls are relatively dry and/or glistening, healing may be enhanced by intramarrow penetration to encourage bleeding and allow the ingress of reparative cells, vessels, and other tissues. Such penetrations can be accomplished with a small round bur or hand instruments.

**7. Use of presuturing.** Loose placement of sutures, left untied, prior to the filling of the defect reduces the possibility that the graft material will be displaced during the suturing process. It also simplifies the last steps of the procedure because once defect fill has been completed, the already placed sutures need only be tied to complete the surgical procedure (Fig 6-2c).

**8. Adequate condensation of graft materials.** The commercial availability of alloplastic materials eliminates the problem of not having enough graft material. The

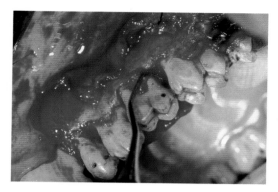

Fig 6-2a  Vertical releasing incisions used to allow proper access to the defects.

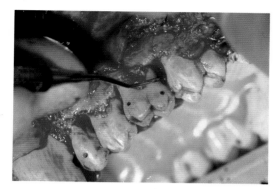

Fig 6-2b  Removal of granulomatous soft tissues from defect and root preparation.

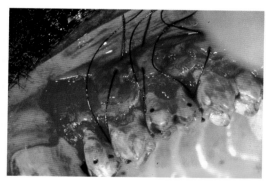

Fig 6-2c  Loose placement of sutures, left untied, prior to the filling of the defect.

graft material should be placed in small increments (Fig 6-2d). Useful in this regard are sterile plastic or polytetrafluoroethylene-lined amalgam carriers to place the material, and sterile amalgam squeeze cloths to use over the suction tip to dry the defect without removing any of the graft material. Small increments of material should be placed in the defect, gently packed into the angles and base of the defect with small pluggers or curets, and dried with the squeeze-cloth–covered suc-

tion tip. The process is repeated until the defect is filled (Fig 6-2e).

**9. Filling to a realistic level.** Except in unusual circumstances, defects should be filled with the synthetic graft materials only to the level of the defect walls. There is little suggestion that overfilling with these materials routinely results in supracrestal bone formation. Overfilling may actually be counterproductive, because it may preclude proper flap closure, thereby retarding healing and possibly resulting in loss of the graft material.

**10. Achievement of good tissue coverage.** A good flap design (see item 3) usually allows primary closure with replaced flaps and contact of the interproximal papillae (Fig 6-2f). If tissue coverage of the ceramic graft material is not satisfactory, additional releasing incisions or reflection may be necessary. Another possible treatment is the use of an autogenous free gingival graft or a freeze-dried skin or dura mater allograft to cover the bone graft site.

**11. Placement of a periodontal dressing.** The use of firm, protective periodontal dressings for 10 days after bone graft surgery is suggested. Placement of an antibiotic ointment under the dressing to help

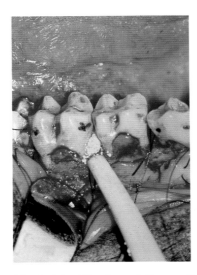

Fig 6-2d   Placing of the graft material in small increments.

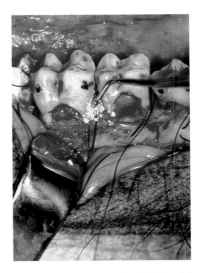

Fig 6-2e   Defect is filled with graft material.

seal the area may be useful. It has become popular not to use dressings after many periodontal surgical procedures, but the possibility of impingement of foreign materials into the graft site, flap displacement, and loss of graft material, any of which would jeopardize the success of treatment, makes the use of protective dressings prudent.

**12. Administration of antibiotics.** A growing body of research data lends support to empirical clinical use of antibiotics peri-surgically when bone grafts are used. Tetracycline-type drugs are the antibiotics of choice for immediate postsurgical plaque suppression because of their broad spectrum of activity, attraction to healing wound sites, and concentration in gingival crevicular fluid. They are administered in therapeutic doses for the first 10 days after surgery or until the patient can practice proper plaque control in the area.

**13. Provision of postsurgical care.** If the dressing and sutures are removed before 10 days, another dressing is often indicated. When the first postoperative

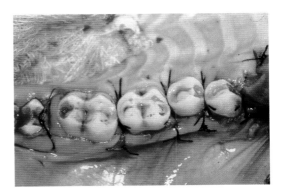

Fig 6-2f   Primary closure with replaced flaps and contact of the interproximal papillae.

treatment occurs 10 or more days after surgery, additional dressings are rarely indicated. The patient should be started immediately on gentle but thorough plaque control methods, including the use of antibacterial rinses, and should be scheduled for professional plaque control in the office as follows: *(1)* every 10 days for three visits, *(2)* every month for two visits, and

109

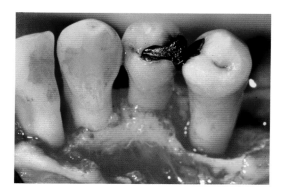

Figs 6-3a to 3c   Clinical result with solid hydroxyapatite bone replacement on mandibular second premolar of a 62-year-old man.

Fig 6-3a   Surgical exposure and debridement of defect and tooth.

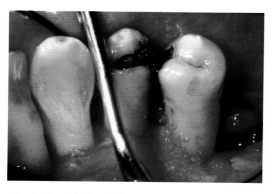

Fig 6-3b   Defect filled to margins with graft material.

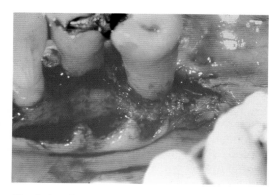

Fig 6-3c Six-month reentry view of repaired defect.

(3) every 3 months, perhaps alternating with the referring dentist. At these visits, a plaque score is taken and oral hygiene procedures are reviewed with, demonstrated to, and practiced by the patient. The patient is rendered plaque-free by office personnel prior to leaving the office. Occasionally, the grafted area may be lightly curetted to help with debridement and to retard epithelial downgrowth. The grafted areas should not be probed before 3 months postsurgically. Also, radiographs taken before 6 months postsurgery provide equivocal information.

# Results using synthetic graft materials

Manufacturer-generated and independent research reports on synthetic ceramic graft materials have consistently demonstrated positive clinical results similar in magnitude and frequency to those obtained with other graft materials. A mean defect fill of about 60% to 70% has been shown with all the materials listed in Table 6-1 with no essential difference between them. The research reports also show that failures occur about

10% of the time. Complete defect fills also occur with about the same frequency. These findings indicate that bone grafting with synthetic materials is not universally successful but does offer the prospect of positive clinical results for the majority of defects in the majority of patients (Evans 1989; Kenney et al 1985; Meffert et al 1985; Rabalais et al 1981; Snyder et al 1984; Strub et al 1979; Yukna et al 1985, 1986). The "partial success" often achieved may be the only treatment needed, or it may allow further therapy such as additional grafting or osseous recontouring to reduce the defect further (Fig 6-3a to c).

The use of bone grafts in periodontics provides the most predictable possibility of regeneration of the entire periodontal attachment apparatus. Additional support for and retention of teeth with substantial vertical bone loss can be achieved. Pocket reduction and growth of alveolar bone have commonly been observed. True histologic new attachment is less frequent and less predictable.

Alloplastic graft materials may have their greatest usefulness as autograft extenders, being added to available autogenous bone to provide a sufficient total volume of graft material. They may also be used as carriers for growth factors, antibiotics, or other substances.

Synthetic bone grafting materials offer promise in periodontal therapy, but they are far from a panacea. They are no better clinically than autogenous or allogenic graft materials. All graft materials make up only one aspect of the treatment of infrabony periodontal defects. More important than the type of graft material is proper patient selection and appropriate surgical management of the defect and the root surface. There is no synthetic substitute for properly performed periodontal surgery.

# References

Becker W, Becker B, Berg L, Prichard J, Caffesse R, Rosenberg E. New attachment after treatment with root isolation procedures. Report for treated Class III and Class II furcations and vertical osseous defects. Int J Periodont Rest Dent 1988; 8(3):9–23.

Boetto J, Freeman E. Histologic evaluation of durapatite in experimental periodontal defects. J Can Dent Assoc 1984;50:239–244.

Bowers GM, Vargo JW, Levy B, Emerson JR, Berquist JJ. Histologic observations following the placement of tricalcium phosphate implants in human intrabony defects. J Periodontol 1986; 57:286–287.

Bowers GM, Chadroff B, Carnevale R, et al. Histologic evaluation of new attachment apparatus formation in humans. Part III. J Periodontol 1989; 60:683–693.

Dragoo MR, Sullivan HC. A clinical and histological evaluation of autogenous iliac bone grafts in humans. Part I. Wound healing 2 to 8 months. J Periodontol 1973;44:599–613.

Evans GH, Yukna RA, Sepe WW, Mabry TW, Mayer ET. Effect of various graft materials with tetracycline in localized juvenile periodontitis. J Periodontol 1989;60:491–497.

Froum SJ, Thaler R, Scopp IW, Stahl SS. Osseous autografts. I. Clinical responses to bone blend or hip marrow grafts. J Periodontol 1975;46:515–521.

Froum SJ, Kushner L, Scopp IW, Stahl SS. Human clinical and histologic responses to durapatite implants in intraosseous lesions. Case reports. J Periodontol 1982;53:719–725.

Frank RM, Gineste M, Benque EP, Hemmerle J, Duffort JF, Heughebaert M. Etude ultrastructurale de l'induction osseuse apres implantation de bioapatites chezl'homme. J Biol Buccale 1987;15: 125–135.

Gottlow J, Nyman S, Lindhe J, Karring T, Wennström J. New attachment formation in the human periodontium by guided tissue regeneration. Case reports. J Clin Periodontol 1986;13:604–616.

Hiatt WH, Schallhorn RG. Intraoral transplants of cancellous bone and marrow in periodontal lesions. J Periodontol 1973;44:194.

Jarcho MJ. Calcium phosphate ceramics as hard tissue prosthetics. Clin Orthop 1981;157:259.

Kenney EB, Lekovic V, Han T, Carranza FA Jr, Dimitrijevic B. The use of a porous hydroxylapatite implant in periodontal defects. J Periodontol 1985; 56:82–88.

Meffert RM, Thomas JR, Hamilton KM, Brownstein CN. Hydroxyapatite as an alloplastic graft in the treatment of human periodontal osseous defects. J Periodontol 1985;56:63–73.

Meffert RM, Thomas JR, Caudill RF. Hydroxyapatite implantation—Clinical and histologic analysis of a treated lesion and speculations regarding healing phenomena. Int J Periodont Rest Dent 1986; 6(6):61–66.

Mellonig JT. Bone grafts and restorative dentistry. In: Malone WFP, Porter ZC, eds. *Tissue Management in Restorative Dentistry.* Boston: Wright, 1982:161–216.

Mellonig JT. Decalcified freeze-dried bone allograft as an implant material in human periodontal defects. *Int J Periodont Rest Dent* 1984;4(6):41–55.

Nabers CL, Reed OM, Hammer JE. Gross and histologic evaluation of an autogenous bone graft 57 months postoperatively. *J Periodontol* 1972;43:702.

Rabalais ML Jr, Yukna RA, Mayer ET. Evaluation of durapatite ceramic as an alloplastic implant in periodontal osseous defects. I. Initial six-month results. *J Periodontol* 1981;52:680–689.

Ross SE, Cohen DW. The fate of a free osseous tissue autograft: A clinical and histological case report. *Periodontics* 1968;6:145.

Sapkos SW. The use of Periograf in periodontal defects—Histologic findings. *J Periodontol* 1986; 57:7–13.

Schallhorn RG, Hiatt WH, Boyce W. Iliac transplants in periodontal therapy. *J Periodontol* 1970;41:566.

Schallhorn RG. Present status of osseous grafting procedures. *J Periodontol* 1977;48:570–576.

Sepe WW, Bowers GM, Lawarence JJ, Friedlander GE, Koch RW. Clinical evaluation of freeze-dried bone allografts in periodontal osseous defects. Part II. *J Periodontol* 1978;49:9.

Snyder AJ, Levin MP, Cutright DE. Alloplastic implants of tricalcium phosphate ceramic in human periodontal osseous defects. *J Periodontol* 1984;55:273–277.

Strub JR, Gaberthuel TW, Firestone AR. Comparison of tricalcium phosphate and frozen allogenic bone implants in man. *J Periodontol* 1979; 50:624–629.

Yukna RA, Harrison BG, Caudill RF, Evans GH, Mayer ET, Miller S. Evaluation of durapatite ceramic as an alloplastic implant in periodontal osseous defects. II. Twelve-month reentry results. *J Periodontol* 1985;56:540–547.

Yukna RA, Cassingham RJ, Caudill RF, et al. Six month evaluation of Calcitite (hydroxyapatite ceramic) in periodontal osseous defects. *Int J Periodont Rest Dent* 1986;6(3):35–45.

Zaner DJ, Yukna RA. Particle size of periodontal bone grafting materials. *J Periodontol* 1984;55: 406–409.

Chapter 7

# Clinical and Histologic Results of Regenerative Procedures

Raul G. Caffesse / Carlos E. Nasjleti

The ultimate goal of periodontal therapy includes the arrest of progressive periodontal disease and the restitution of those parts of the periodontium that were destroyed by the disease (Kalkwarf 1974; Stahl 1977). Another goal of therapy is predictable regeneration of the periodontium at the site of previous breakdown. Periodontal regeneration relates to forming new periodontal connective tissue components (cementum, periodontal ligament, and alveolar bone) from a reduced periodontium, and obtaining deposition of the new cementum on the periodontally exposed root surface (Polson and Caton 1982).

## New attachment procedures

Traditionally, the accepted surgical techniques used for connective tissue reattachment have been subgingival curettage (Goldman 1949), the modified Widman flap procedure (Ramfjord and Nissle 1974), and various modifications of these two basic procedures. Both techniques have been thoroughly studied and evaluated

(Knowles et al 1979; Ramfjord et al 1975; Zamet 1975). In clinical studies, use of the modified Widman flap procedure has resulted in closure of infrabony pockets, gain in probing attachment level, and minimal bone resorption (Rosling et al 1976). However, histologic studies showed that minimal or no attachment is achieved, and that the rest of the marginal seal is established by a long junctional epithelium (Caton et al 1980; Steiner et al 1981).

## Grafting materials

In a number of studies, the flap procedure has been combined with insertion of different kinds of bone and ceramic grafts into the curetted bony defects to achieve new attachment.

### Bone grafts

Many studies have shown an increased bone fill with the use of bone grafts, including autografts, allografts, and xenografts (Bowen et al 1989; Dragoo 1981; Ellegaard et al 1976a; Froum et al 1976;

Hiatt and Schallhorn 1973; Mellonig 1984; Rummelhart et al 1989), and it has been postulated that new attachment occurs where new bone is present. In general, clinical parameters such as probing depth, attachment level, and radiographic bone height show significant improvement and are considered to represent evidence of new attachment.

However, caution has been exercised in accepting the absolute value of clinical measurements made in these bone graft studies. Gara and Adams (1981) summarize the opinions of some investigators in the following statement:

> Not one of the human implant studies to date has provided the type of experimental model that clearly demonstrates new attachment formation. Many of the investigators have failed to provide controls, and none have provided the unequivocal histologic evidence of new attachment to previously diseased root surface.

Egelberg (1987) stated that there is

> ... little indication that grafts of cortical or cancellous bone have any inductive effect on the formation of new bone. Further, there is little reason to believe that such bone grafts would stimulate connective tissue attachment to root surface.

Others have also questioned the value of bone grafts and whether or not a graft contributes to new attachment (Caton et al 1980; Gantes et al 1988; Listgarten and Rosenberg 1979; Martin et al 1988; Moskow et al 1979; Steiner et al 1981).

Recently, however, Bowers et al (1989a, 1989b) presented histologic evidence of new attachment apparatus following placement of a decalcified freeze-dried bone allograft in intrabony defects, both in a submerged and nonsubmerged environ-

ment in humans. For these studies, grafted and nongrafted sites were histometrically evaluated and compared 6 months after surgery. Results indicated that significantly more new attachment apparatus, including cementum, bone, and periodontal ligament, forms in intrabony defects that are grafted with demineralized bone than in nongrafted defects.

**Ceramic grafts**

Grafts of ceramic tricalcium phosphate and hydroxyapatite, including a porous hydroxyapatite of coral origin, have been evaluated (Bowen et al 1989; Bowers et al 1986; Froum et al 1982; Kenney et al 1986; Meffert et al 1985; Yukna et al 1984). In these studies, bone formation around grafted particles was reported but may not occur regularly. The beneficial effects of these grafts over bone grafts or nongraft procedures has not been convincingly demonstrated (Egelberg 1987). However, their use as a "filler" in specific situations may need to be explored further (Egelberg 1987).

# Citric acid root conditioning

Histologic evidence of cementogenesis and new connective tissue attachment to previously diseased root surfaces, with the use of citric acid demineralization, has been reported in animal studies (Cole et al 1980; Nilveus et al 1980; Register and Burdick 1976). Although several animal studies have shown that this treatment facilitates attachment of connective tissue to root surfaces, clinical studies have failed to demonstrate that citric acid is a significant adjuvant to surgical debridement (Albair et al 1982; Renvert and Egelberg 1981; Renvert et al 1985; Smith et al 1986; Stahl and Froum 1977). Albair et al (1982) concluded that, although a functionally oriented connective tissue attachment is established with the citric acid conditioning of root surfaces, the predictability of the process is questionable. Furthermore, the initial healing observed after citric acid demineralization is often hampered by irreversible resorption and ankylosis of the root (Magnusson et al 1985a; Pettersson and Aukhil 1986; Wikesjö et al 1988).

Gantes et al (1988) treated a total of 30 mandibular buccal class II furcation defects in 22 subjects using a regenerative surgical therapy that included citric acid conditioning and coronally positioned flaps secured by crown-attached sutures (Klinge et al 1981, 1985; Martin et al 1988). In addition, grafts of freeze-dried, decalcified allogenic bone were placed in 16 of the 30 defects. The effect of the treatments was evaluated from a series of soft and hard tissue measurements. These measurements demonstrated notable improvements 12 months after therapy. On the average, 67% of the defect volume became filled with bone, and 43% of treated defects were completely closed by bone fill. No difference was observed between defects treated with and without bone grafts.

## Tetracycline root conditioning

Tetracycline has also been used in regenerative periodontal procedures. Many types of bacteria found in periodontal diseases are susceptible to tetracycline (Baker et al 1983; Bjorvatn et al 1984; Walker et al 1985). In the periodontal wound area, tetracyclines may act to reduce gingival collagenolytic activity (Ericsson et al 1987; Golub et al 1985), increase fibroblastic attachment and spreading on the root surface (Somerman et al 1988; Terranova et al 1987), decrease epithelial cell attachment (Terranova et al 1986), and etch the dentin

surface (Wikesjö et al 1986). In this last study, tetracycline hydrochloride conditioning removed the smear layer, thereby exposing dentin with open tubules. Hence, Terranova et al (1986) and Wikesjö et al (1986) suggested that root surface conditioning with tetracycline hydrochloride may facilitate healing of the hard tissue–soft tissue interface. This improved healing may result from the provision of a suitable root surface as substrate for mesenchymal cells and from the antimicrobial activity of the antibiotic.

Frantz and Polson (1988) evaluated tissue interactions to dentin demineralized with different concentrations of tetracycline solutions (200 mg/cm$^3$ or 100 mg/cm$^3$) for 5 minutes. Dentin specimens were obtained from beneath root surfaces covered by periodontal ligament. Dentin specimens were implanted transcutaneously into incisional wounds on the dorsal surface of rats with one end protruding through the skin. They were available for histologic and histometric analysis 1 and 10 days after implantation. Tetracycline-treated surfaces had greater numbers of attached cells at both time points compared to untreated controls. No differences were discernible related to different tetracycline concentrations. The authors concluded that tetracycline-demineralized dentin provides a substrate that increases cell attachment; however, this enhanced response does not result in a connective tissue attachment.

Claffey et al (1987) tested the effect of topically applied tetracycline on healing subsequent to periodontal surgery. For this study, the alveolar bone around mandibular premolars was surgically reduced up to 6 mm from the cementoenamel junction in two beagle dogs. The denuded root surfaces were exposed to the oral environment during 3 months without plaque control. Regenerative surgery was then carried out, using root surface conditioning with 1% tetracycline and coronally repositioned

115

flaps. Six months later, histologic evaluation showed connective tissue attachment extending to the cementoenamel junction in most of the specimens. However, superficial root resorption was prevalent in the cervical region. Apical to this region, an area of ankylosis was present in most specimens. In some instances ankylosis had been preceded by superficial root resorption. Histologic examination also showed that ankylosis was prevalent in the fornix of the furcations.

Wikesjö et al (1988) examined the repair of periodontal furcation defects in beagle dogs following reconstructive surgery that included root surface demineralization with tetracycline hydrochloride and topical fibronectin application. In 14 beagle dogs, horizontal periodontal defects were surgically induced around the mandibular premolars, followed by 6 weeks without plaque control. Reconstructive surgery of the defects was subsequently carried out. The root surfaces were debrided and conditioned with citric acid or tetracycline hydrochloride, with or without subsequent application of fibronectin. The animals were killed 12 weeks after surgery. Histologically, the study showed that: *(1)* citric acid conditioning of the root surface frequently results in complete connective tissue repair of the furcation defect; *(2)* root resorption and ankylosis are prevalent features of the healing response; *(3)* citric acid and tetracycline treatment have similar potential to induce connective tissue repair and result in corresponding incidences of root resorption and ankylosis; and *(4)* application of fibronectin to demineralized root surfaces does not enhance the amount of connective tissue repair and does not alter the pattern of root resorption and ankylosis.

Clearly, additional investigations are indicated to determine the place of root surface conditioning with tetracycline in periodontal tissue regeneration procedures.

# Fibronectin

Specific attachment glycoproteins (Fernyhough and Page 1983; Terranova and Martin 1982) and plasma factors may be the essential substrata for the basic cellular and molecular interactions between fibroblasts and root surfaces. An ingredient of whole blood that appears to offer potential for retarding epithelial downgrowth is the noncollagenous glycoprotein, *fibronectin*. Fibronectin is a major participant in a variety of cellular activities such as cell-cell and cell-substrate adhesiveness (Pearlstein 1976; Yamada and Weston 1974), cell spreading, locomotion, and morphology (Ali et al 1977; Yamada et al 1978). These adhesive functions are brought about or are at least partially modulated by the binding and cross-linking of fibronectin to certain extracellular macromolecules such as collagen, fibrinogen, and/or fibrin (Kleinman et al 1981; Ruoslahti and Vaheri 1975; Yamada et al 1985). Related studies indicate that fibronectin performs several functions involved in the body's response to injury during wound healing, clot formation, and hemostasis (Bitterman et al 1983; Kurkinen et al 1980; Pommier et al 1983). These activities have led to attempts to use fibronectin to foster the reattachment of periodontal tissues to the root surface in the surgical treatment of periodontal disease (Caffesse et al 1985, 1987; Nasjleti et al 1986, 1987; Terranova and Martin 1982).

Recent work involving fibronectin has opened new avenues with respect to the treatment of exposed root surfaces and, in particular, furcation defects. Weiss and Reddi (1981) have shown in animal models that the physiologic role of fibronectin in tissue morphogenesis is to allow for initial extracellular matrix-cell attachment. Grinnell and Bennett (1981) have shown in vitro that fibronectin is probably necessary for fibroblast adhesion and connective tissue organization in healing wounds.

116

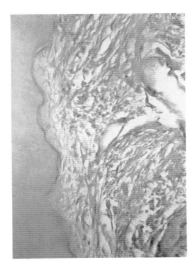 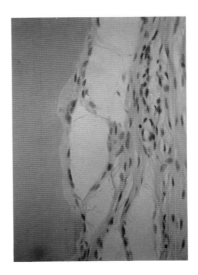

Fig 7-1a   *(Left)* Beagle dog specimen with natural periodontitis. The area was treated with citric acid demineralization and fibronectin application. Observe the attachment of connective tissue fibers to the root surface. (Hematoxylin and eosin stain; original magnification × 35.)

Fig 7-1b   *(Right)* Area similar to that in Fig 7-1a at higher magnification to show the fiber reattachment to the root in an area that was previously exposed to the periodontal pocket. (Hematoxylin and eosin stain; original magnification × 100.)

Fernyhough and Page (1983) demonstrated greatly enhanced cell attachment of fibroblasts to both normal and periodontally diseased roots following root planing and pretreatment with fibronectin. Wikesjö et al (1986) described a biochemical approach to improve new connective tissue attachment by treatment of dentin surfaces with tetracycline and application of fibronectin. They showed that the attachment and growth of gingival fibroblasts and gingival epithelial cells on dentin surfaces prepared with tetracycline hydrochloride can be modulated by laminin and fibronectin (Terranova et al 1986). Further, conditioned dentin surfaces that are subsequently treated with fibronectin act as poor substrates for the attachment and proliferation of gingival epithelial cells.

Caffesse et al (1985) determined the effect of citric acid conditioning and fibronectin application on healing following surgical treatment of naturally occurring periodontal disease in beagle dogs. Significantly increased amounts of connective tissue reattachment are observed in the areas treated with the citric acid and fibronectin combination (Figs 7-1a and b). Fibrous reattachment is enhanced at the expense of epithelial downgrowth and occurs directly to both new and old cementum and exposed dentin, often in a functional manner (ie, perpendicular to the root surface).

Subsequently, Smith et al (1987a) determined the effects of citric acid and fibronectin and laminin application in treating periodontitis in beagle dogs. For the study, all four quadrants in each dog were used. Each quadrant included the premolars and first molar teeth. Two treatments were used and were comparatively analyzed for differences in histologic healing responses 120

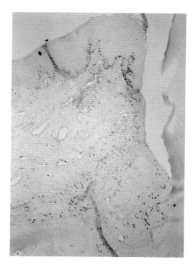

Fig 7-2a   Rhesus monkey specimen treated with citric acid and fibronectin. Tritiated thymidine labeling shows significant cellular proliferation of the supracrestal tissues. Specimen at 7 days. (Hematoxylin and eosin stain; original magnification × 25.)

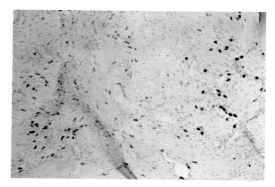

Fig 7-2b   Higher magnification of Fig 7-2a that clearly depicts the labeling uptake in the supracrestal connective tissues. (Hematoxylin and eosin stain; original magnification × 64.)

days after surgery. The treatments were: (1) surgery (mucoperiosteal flaps) plus citric acid and (2) surgery plus citric acid followed by fibronectin-laminin application. When laminin was used in addition to citric acid and fibronectin, there were no im-

provements of results beyond those obtained with the use of citric acid alone, although fibronectin was also applied. As a consequence, the result was a long junctional epithelium that reached the coronal border of the root notches.

Caffesse et al (1987) evaluated histologically and autoradiographically the effects of citric acid conditioning and autologous fibronectin application on cell proliferation after mucoperiosteal flap surgery. Three adult rhesus monkeys were used for the study. Surgeries were staggered to produce the following time periods: 3, 7, 15, 21, and 28 days. Fibronectin-treated areas showed significantly increased cellular proliferation during the first 2 weeks, with all the supracrestal tissues being affected, and it was concluded that application of citric acid followed by fibronectin enhances cellular proliferation (Figs 7-2a and b). Following this publication, Smith et al (1987b) reported on the effect of citric acid and various concentrations of fibronectin on healing after periodontal flap surgery in dogs. Exogenous fibronectin in increasing concentrations (0.38, 0.75, and 1.5 mg/mL of saline) was used. There was a significant increase in new connective attachment in all surgical sites where fibronectin had been added (Fig 7-3), but there was no obvious advantage in increasing the concentration of fibronectin above the plasma level (0.38 mg/mL).

Caffesse et al (1988a) reported clinical results of the use of citric acid and autologous fibronectin. The study population comprised 29 patients under treatment for moderate to advanced periodontitis who reached the 1-year posttherapy evaluation. The evaluation indicated that both approaches used—modified Widman flap alone or in combination with citric acid and fibronectin—significantly reduce probing pocket depth and increase clinical attachment (Figs 7-4 and 7-5). However, the changes achieved with citric acid and fibro-

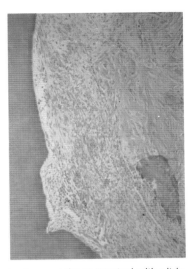

Fig 7-3 Beagle dog specimen treated with citric acid and plasma concentration of fibronectin. Observe the reattachment of the connective tissues to the root surface. (Hematoxylin and eosin stain; original magnification × 50.)

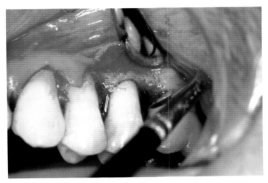

Fig 7-4 Clinical application of citric acid after modified Widman flap reflection, thorough root planing, and debridement. The citric acid (pH 1) is applied with a camel's hair brush for 3 minutes.

nectin were statistically greater than those obtained with the flap procedure alone. Furthermore, the number of sites that gained 2 mm or more of clinical attachment increased significantly.

Peltzman et al (1988) reported clinical observations following treatment of furcation involvements with fibronectin and intraoral autogenous bone grafts. Four patients with buccal furcation involvement on bilateral mandibular molars were selected for the study. A mucoperiosteal flap was reflected to gain access to the defects. Bone obtained from the surgical site was mixed with the patient's plasma fibronectin in a dappen dish. Furcation sites that received the mixture of bone and fibronectin (experimental) were selected by alternating defect design. After 6 months, there were some differences in attachment gain and clinical probing depths favoring those furcation sites treated with the autogenous bone–fibronectin blend. However, the differences were slight and there were so few

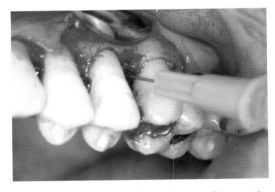

Fig 7-5 Application of autologous fibronectin after citric acid conditioning and thorough rinsing. The fibronectin is applied with a tuberculin syringe.

defects that comparison may be misleading. Furthermore, no bone fill was recorded in any of the experimental or control sites.

More recently, a follow-up report evaluated 46 patients 1 year after treatment and reported significant gains in clinical attachment and probing depth reduction when citric acid and fibronectin were used (Caffesse et al 1990a). Two-year follow-up reviews in 26 patients showed insignificant difference in probing depth reductions while the significant improvement in clinical attachment was still maintained.

Thus, there have been encouraging results associated with citric acid conditioning and subsequent fibronectin application on root surfaces. Additional clinical investigations are indicated to determine the place of this treatment combination in periodontal therapy.

# Growth factors

Growth factors are naturally occurring polypeptide molecules, somewhat like hormones in structure and function, but they exert potent *local activity* rather than a systemic effect. These substances are a class of natural biologic mediators that regulate the proliferation, differentiation, motility, and matrix synthesis of nearly all cell types (Terranova and Wikesjö 1987; Wirthlin 1989). These properties, demonstrable in vitro, have led to the proposal that such factors play important roles in soft and hard tissue repair.

Terranova et al (1987) reported that fibronectin and endothelial cell growth factor can contribute to periodontal regeneration by inducing attachment, migration, and proliferation of periodontal ligament cells. Subsequently, Terranova et al (1989) reported data that indicated basic fibroblast growth factor can stimulate periodontal ligament and human endothelial cell migration as well as human endothelial cell proliferation. Further, these authors showed that basic fibroblastic growth factor binding is increased by the exposure of type I collagen in dentin.

Lynch et al (1987) showed that platelet-derived growth factor (PDGF) and insulin-like growth factor (IGF-1) interact synergis-

tically to accelerate the healing of partial-thickness porcine skin wounds. Topical application of the PDGF–IGF-1 combination stimulated increased DNA, collagen, and noncollagenous protein synthesis, which resulted in a doubling of connective tissue volume within the wound during the first week of healing. This report was followed by another (Lynch et al 1989) that showed that a combination of PDGF and IGF-1 enhances periodontal regeneration. For the study, the combination of growth factors was applied to periodontitis-affected teeth in beagle dogs. One microgram of PDGF and IGF-1 in an aqueous gel was applied to the root surfaces of test teeth following open flap debridement. Control sites received the gel alone. Two weeks after treatment, histologic analysis of control specimens revealed a long junctional epithelial attachment and no new bone or cementum formation. In contrast, growth factor–treated sites exhibited significant amounts of new bone and cementum formation. The authors postulated that, because both PDGF and IGF-1 have been shown to be potent mitogens and chemotactic agents for both fibroblasts and osteoblasts when applied in vivo, they may stimulate migration of these cells into the area, as well as promote their proliferation. Furthermore, these growth factors appear to be capable of stimulating metabolic processes of the recruited cells, leading to new collagen and bone formation.

Certainly, the above initial observations indicate that biologic growth factors may have significant potential for periodontal regeneration. Additional studies should be encouraged.

# Membranes

Nyman et al (1982a, 1982b) were the first to use a barrier or membrane in periodontal healing studies. They reported that partial regeneration of periodontal tissues was

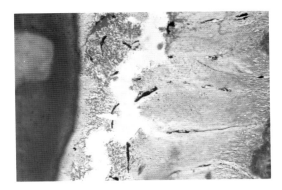

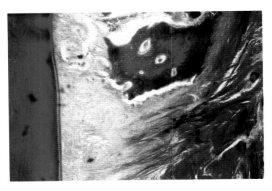

Fig 7-6　Rhesus monkey tooth 3 days after replantation. Although tissues attached to the tooth do not show vascular patency (lack of India ink perfusion), they protect the root and favor reattachment of the tissues. (Mallory's stain; original magnification × 40.)

Fig 7-7　Monkey tooth 15 days after replantation, where remaining periodontal tissues were preserved. Observe complete healing of the periodontal ligament and lack of maturation of healed tissues. (Mallory's stain; original magnification × 40.)

obtained when a Millipore filter (Millipore, Bedford, MA) was interposed between the gingival tissue on one side and the exposed root surface and the surrounding alveolar bone on the other. The role of the Millipore filter was twofold: first, to serve as a barrier against the colonization of the exposed root surface by gingival cells; second, to allow selective repopulation of this surface by periodontal ligament cells, on the theory that progenitor cells arising from the periodontal ligament are the only ones with the potential to differentiate into cementoblasts. This coronal periodontal cell proliferation implies that the proliferation of other tissues must be blocked. This current concept evolved from a large number of previous studies on periodontal tissue healing. The following brief review highlights the studies that have contributed to the understanding that periodontal ligament cells are necessary for new attachment formation and describes current techniques being used to attain the selective repopulation of the root surface by periodontal ligament cells.

The importance of the periodontal ligament as basic in regenerative procedures was shown by Löe and Waerhaug (1961). They conducted long-term experiments in which they intentionally replanted teeth in dogs and monkeys; their studies showed that replanted teeth with vital periodontal ligament always show reformation of the attachment apparatus. The authors sustained the concept that successful replantation of teeth depends on the maintenance of a viable periodontal ligament. Their view was shared by many investigators, including Nasjleti et al (1975a, 1975b), Andreasen (1981), and Proye and Polson (1982a, 1982b). These studies, however, did not consider the role of other components of the periodontium, including epithelial migration, during healing (Figs 7-6 and 7-7).

Björn blamed the absence of new attachment on epithelial migration along the root surface (Björn 1961; Björn et al 1965) and suggested that if total exclusion of the epithelium were possible, complete regeneration of the attachment apparatus could occur. To accomplish this, Björn and coworkers cut off the crown of periodontally treated teeth and covered the stump completely with a mucosal flap. Because the healing epithelium was distant from the root surface, no epithelial migration took place. The study demonstrated that new attachment formation is not produced merely by epithelial exclusion, and that neither bone nor gingival connective tissue can produce new attachment on a root surface from which the periodontal ligament tissue is absent.

Ellegaard et al (1974, 1976b) carried out a differently designed study. They covered the flap margins with a free gingival graft, working on the premise that because the surface epithelium of a free gingival graft initially degenerates and then regenerates during healing, they would have about 10 to 14 days for connective tissue to reattach to the root before epithelium migrated downward to prevent this attachment. Although there was some success with these procedures, predictability was a problem.

Nyman et al (1980) tested Björn's hypothesis by developing an experimental model in which the epithelium was excluded from the healing process. In that model, periodontitis-affected roots were planed and sectioned from their crowns. The roots were then longitudinally embedded to half their width in a trough made in alveolar bone and then covered with a mucoperiosteal flap. Each embedded root was therefore allowed to heal without the influence of the epithelium. Four different healing zones were seen: those adjacent to bone with and without intact periodontal ligament tissue, and those adjacent to gingival connective tissue with and without intact periodontal ligament tissue. The study confirmed other studies that suggested that epithelial exclusion and periodontal ligament tissue are necessary for new attachment (Karring et al 1980; Line et al 1974; Melcher 1970). Another finding of this study was that on denuded root surfaces gingival connective tissue causes root resorption and bone causes ankylosis. These findings agreed with those of other

studies (Andreasen 1976; Andreasen and Kristerson 1981), but it was not known whether this resorption and failure to obtain new attachment was caused by the inability of these tissues to produce new attachment, or if the *diseased* root surface was biologically incompatible and was being resorbed because of its toxicity (Aleo et al 1975).

Karring et al (1980) implanted thoroughly planed periodontitis-affected roots into surgically created sockets in edentulous areas to exclude epithelial migration and infection. The apical areas previously unexposed to disease showed new cementum formation with collagen fibers functionally oriented along the root. Despite the absence of epithelium, the coronal area previously exposed to disease had no new fibrous attachment. Instead, repair occurred by resorption and ankylosis. When gingival connective tissue was allowed to come in contact with a denuded root surface, it produced resorption, whereas bone produced ankylosis. These findings corroborated those of others (Andreasen 1976, 1981; Line et al 1974; Melcher 1976) and were interpreted to mean that bone cells migrate to contact the root during healing and are responsible for the changes that took place.

Considering such findings, it was surprising that treatment of infrabony defects by grafting did not result in resorption and ankylosis. Karring et al (1980) postulated that the apical proliferation of the junctional epithelium may be one reason that resorption infrequently takes place. An epithelial barrier that forms before granulation tissue from the alveolar bone can reach the root surface may prevent this repair process from taking place. When the epithelium is prevented from reaching the infrabony defect during healing, root resorption is common (Björn et al 1965).

Andreasen (1981) demonstrated that root resorption may also be prevented by the presence of a periodontal ligament. He extracted incisors and removed a circular area of periodontal ligament tissue from each of these teeth. He either left this circular area uncovered or covered it with one of seven periodontal ligament substitutes: cultured periodontal ligament cells; dental follicle cells; fascia; gingival, mucosal, or cutaneous connective tissue; or periosteum. The uncovered areas resorbed, whereas the substitutes greatly or partially prevented resorption. Only the periodontal ligament cells and dental follicle greatly reduced resorption and produced new cementum.

In a similar study in dogs, periodontal ligament cells were cultured and placed on planed root surfaces. These were then implanted on surgically created troughs in dogs and compared to planed root surfaces either colonized by gingival connective tissue cells or left uncovered as controls. Only those colonized by periodontal ligament cells produced new attachment. Resorption and ankylosis were prominent features of the other teeth (Boyko et al 1981).

Hence, the aforementioned studies suggested that new connective tissue attachment can be achieved on previously diseased roots in both humans and animals, provided that the cells that repopulate the healing root surface are of the proper origin and potential. Melcher (1976) suggested that during healing, the root surface may be repopulated by cells from any of these four sources: epithelium, gingival connective tissue, periodontal ligament, and bone. The periodontal ligament cells are further responsible for maintaining the integrity of fibers, bone, and cementum. Melcher also postulated that during healing, the cells that repopulate the wound determine the nature of the attachment. As shown by other investigators (Andreasen and Hjorting-Hansen 1966; Line et al 1974), if the periodontal wound is colonized by bone cells, ankylosis takes place as new bone comes in contact with the root surface. Melcher (1976) further postulated that "if surgical procedures could be designed such that both periodontal ligament and bone would be allowed to migrate coronally, then cells with the capacity to regenerate and maintain the periodontium would colonize the wound." He suggested that colonization of the root surface by any cell other than the periodontal ligament cell will prevent the formation of new attachment and such colonization must be avoided when surgical techniques aimed at new attachment are designed.

Although there is little doubt that the periodontal ligament is the ideal source of cells for new attachment, to date it has not been conclusively shown that other connective tissues lack the potential for promoting regeneration (Heaney 1986). McHugh (1988) evaluated the effects of exclusion of epithelium from healing periodontal pockets. Results of the study suggested that, although most new attachment appears to result from cells originating in the periodontal ligament, it could also arise from cells from the gingival connective tissue. Melcher et al (1986) and McCulloch et al (1987) have indicated the possibility of cementum deposition as a consequence of proliferation that originates from bone marrow cells.

Nojima et al (1990) examined the possibility that periodontal ligament cells can differentiate into osteoblasts and/or cementoblasts both in freshly isolated periodontal tissues and cultured cells derived from periodontal ligament. Results of the study indicated that the periodontal ligament cells have phenotypes typical of osteoblasts, indicating that they may differentiate into osteoblasts and/or cementoblasts. The authors concluded that periodontal ligament tissues contain cells with several phenotypes of osteoblasts. These findings support the hypothesis that after periodontal therapy, periodontal ligament cells can form a new connective tissue attachment with the newly formed cementum.

## Studies using nonresorbable barriers

As previously mentioned, Nyman et al (1982a, 1982b) introduced an early technique that was intended to prevent colonization of the root surface by epithelium or gingival connective tissue and thereby enhance the repopulation of the root surface by cells derived from the periodontal ligament. A barrier (Millipore filter) was placed between the soft tissue flap and the treated root surface so that the epithelium and gingival connective tissue would be diverted from the root surface. Although this technique did not divert the cells derived from bone, it was thought that the periodontal ligament cells were able to colonize the root surface faster, so the desired result was obtained.

Cementum with inserting connective tissue fibers formed on the curetted portions of the root. Also, significant bone regeneration formed on the test sites. These studies demonstrated that new cementum and new connective tissue attachment could form on root surfaces that have been surgically deprived of their original cementum and periodontal ligament. Although cementum formation was seen in only 50% of the test sites, these studies showed that new attachment, following the principle of guided tissue regeneration, is a strong possibility. Furthermore, because there were no negative effects from the use of such a barrier, the preliminary findings suggested that the placement of a physical barrier between curetted root surfaces and mucoperiosteal flaps might be beneficial in new attachment procedures.

The same principle was applied in a study by Gottlow et al (1984), who worked on three monkeys to test the predictability of controlled tissue regeneration by preventing the epithelium and gingival connective tissue from participating in the healing process. Four teeth in each of the monkeys were used as test units while the contralateral teeth served as controls. The coronal half of the buccal roots was surgically exposed and plaque was allowed to accumulate for 6 months, after which a buccal flap was raised and the roots were planed. The crowns were resected from the roots and the flaps coronally positioned to completely submerge the roots. Before any sutures were placed, however, either a Millipore filter or a Gore-Tex periodontal membrane (an expanded-polytetrafluoroethylene material [WL Gore, Flagstaff, AZ]) was placed over the denuded surface of the test teeth. The results after 3 months of healing showed new cementum with inserting collagen fibers on the previously exposed surfaces of both test and control teeth. However, the test root surfaces exhibited considerably more new attachment, sometimes up to 6.8 mm, indicating that the placement of a membrane favored repopulation of the wound area adjacent to the roots by cells originating from the periodontal ligament. New cementum was always in continuity with the cementum in the unexposed parts and was thicker on the apical part than in the coronal part of the root. Alveolar bone regrowth occurred to a varying extent. This study also demonstrated that new attachment is possible on root surfaces previously exposed to plaque, as shown by other investigators (Bogle et al 1985; Isidor et al 1985; Nyman et al 1982b). This study model made it possible for bone cells to invade the wound area. The only entities that were actually prevented from interfering with healing were gingival connective tissue and epithelium. However, ankylosis was not observed, and it was concluded that granulation tissue from bone does not reach the root faster than granulation tissue from the periodontal ligament. Although test specimens showed root resorption coronal to the new attachment, resorption was more common in the control roots.

The fact that resorption occurred even in test roots implies that gingival connective tissue may have invaded the wound. It was reasonable to assume therefore that the membrane placed on the test sites did not in all instances prevent invasion of the granulation tissue from the gingiva into the space between the membrane and the root. There were no obvious differences with regard to new attachment formation with the use of either the Millipore filter or the Gore-Tex membrane, although cementumlike substances with inserting collagen fibers were occasionally deposited on the surface of the Gore-Tex periodontal material (Gottlow et al 1984). It is possible that the Gore-Tex membrane was more biocompatible than the Millipore filter.

Magnusson et al (1985b) used the Millipore filter in monkeys in a manner similar to that used by Nyman et al (1982a). In essence the membranes were placed between the flap and the roots of human mandibular incisors and remained exposed supragingivally. In the test sites, which received the filter, new attachment was observed to cover approximately 50% of the root surfaces, which previously had been surgically exposed and allowed to accumulate plaque. The control sites healed by a long junctional epithelium and exhibited little or no new attachment. These results showed a considerably lower percentage of new attachment than the study by Gottlow et al (1984), but this may be explained not only by the different filter placement, but also by the fact that the available root length was reduced by the crown resection in Gottlow's design. Root resorption was not found in either the test or control specimens, so the authors concluded that the roots were protected from the gingival connective tissue by a long junctional epithelium in the control sites and by the filter in the test sites.

Because progenitor cells for the formation of connective tissue attachment were believed to be located in the periodontal ligament (Melcher 1976), it was thought that the use of the Millipore filter facilitates repopulation of curetted root surfaces by cells from the periodontal ligament. The barrier creates a "periodontal space" where periodontal cells can migrate coronally, and at the same time it prevents epithelium and gingival connective tissue from contacting the root. However, because evidence was circumstantial and the degree of reported connective tissue formation varied, Aukhil et al (1986a) experimented on multiple teeth of beagle dogs using filters to attempt coronal circumferential migration of cells. Their results showed that while new connective tissue was mostly seen at the apical part of the 8- and 16-week-old specimens, some specimens showed the formation of a long junctional epithelium along the root surface. Those that showed regeneration had up to about 2.94 mm of new attachment formation. Root resorption, which was sometimes seen, preceded the formation of new cementum. These preliminary findings of Aukhil et al suggested that placement of physical barriers between root surfaces and flaps may be beneficial in facilitating coronal migration of progenitor cells from the periodontal ligament. It was suggested, however, that contact between periodontal ligament cells and root dentin is necessary for these progenitor cells to differentiate into formative cells such as cementoblasts (Aukhil et al 1986b). Although it is apparent that periodontal ligament cells induce new attachment via the use of filters, there was no evidence that such physical barriers allow repopulation of curetted root surfaces only from the periodontal ligament. Possibly some cells also originate from the crestal bone covered by the membrane (Aukhil et al 1986a, 1986c).

Caffesse et al (1988b) further tested the Gore-Tex periodontal material on periodontally affected mandibular premolars and first molars of beagle dogs. After raising a

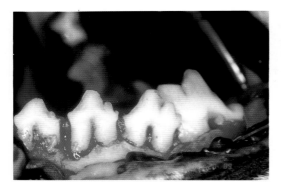

Fig 7-8a A mucoperiosteal flap has been elevated, the area has been debrided, and notches have been placed on each root at the level of the alveolar crest.

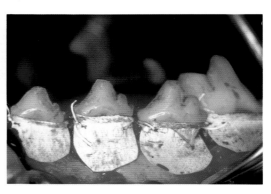

Fig 7-8b Gore-Tex Periodontal Material applied to $P^2$, $P^3$, $P^4$, and $M^1$ on experimental sites.

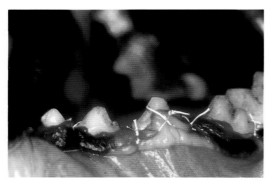

Fig 7-8c The flaps are positioned slightly coronally and sutured. Care was taken to avoid displacement of the periodontal material during the suturing procedure.

mucoperiosteal flap and notching the teeth at the level of the alveolar crest, they applied the membrane on the experimental teeth. The flaps were then positioned slightly coronally and sutured (Figs 7-8a to c). When the membranes were removed, the investigators observed brilliant red granulation tissue that grew from underneath the membrane and was attached to the root. Results showed that although control teeth healed with a long junctional epithelium to the level of the notch, the experimental teeth showed new cementum formation in and even coronal to the notch, with periodontal ligament fibers inserting into the newly formed cementum. Histometric measurements showed significantly greater new attachment formation in the experimental teeth than in the controls. There was no significant difference between sites that retained the membrane for 30 days (mean increase of 1.09 mm), and those that retained it longer (mean of 1.13 mm).

In another study, Caffesse et al (1990c) evaluated the effects of guided tissue regeneration in the treatment of class II furcation defects in six beagle dogs. Gore-Tex periodontal material was used, and the amount of furcation fill and the surface area corresponding to new connective tissue attachment and new bone were evaluated. Results of the study demonstrated different degrees of fill attained by epithelium, new connective tissue, and bone. Statistically, guided tissue regeneration gave significantly better results in the amount of connective tissue and bone fill achieved (Figs 7-9a to d).

Gottlow et al (1986) published another report on new attachment formation, this time on 10 human subjects and using Gore-Tex membranes alone. They assessed the predictability of such formation when the

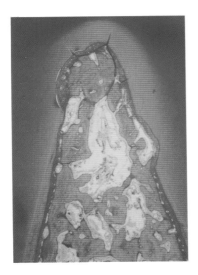 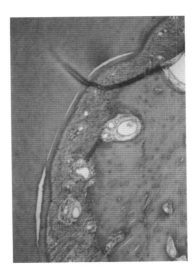

Fig 7-9a *(Left)* Low-power view of a furcation treated with Gore-Tex. Significant amounts of new bone are coronal to reference notches and new attachment is present without evidence of dentoalveolar ankylosis. (Hematoxylin and eosin stain; original magnification × 10.)

Fig 7-9b *(Right)* A higher-power view of an area of Fig 7-9a showing new cementum, bone, and connective tissue fiber arrangement. (Hematoxylin and eosin stain; original magnification × 64.)

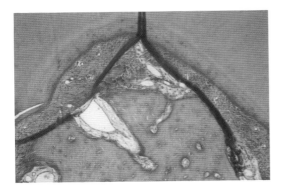

Fig 7-9c A higher-power view of the furcation fornix of Fig 7-9a showing new connective tissue fibers between the new bone and the tooth. (Hematoxylin and eosin stain; original magnification × 64.)

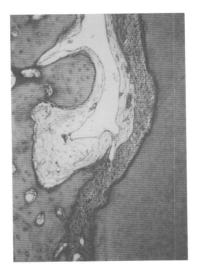

Fig 7-9d A higher-power view of another area of Fig 7-9a showing formation of new bone and new attachment. However, minor amounts of arrested root resorption are evident in the area of the notch. (Hematoxylin and eosin stain; original magnification × 64.)

principles of guided tissue regeneration were applied. For the study, they used 12 teeth with advanced periodontitis from various locations in the mouth. After treatment, five of the teeth, one of which was treated without the membrane, were removed en bloc for histologic analysis. The remaining seven teeth were allowed to remain and were evaluated clinically for success. Eleven teeth, documented as case reports, showed a large variation in the amount of new attachment formed. Histologically, new bone growth seemed to be restricted to areas that had infrabony lesions prior to treatment. Bone regrowth and new attachment appeared to be unrelated phenomena. The authors attributed this variation to variables such as the amount of recession, the type of defect, and the availability of periodontal ligament cells, but they concluded that much work remains regarding predictability.

Also in humans, Pontoriero et al (1988), in compliance with the principles of guided tissue regeneration and using the Gore-Tex periodontal material, treated class II furcation defects. They reported that at most sites it resulted in the disappearance of the anatomic defect. More than 90% of the sites treated with the procedure showed complete resolution of the furcation problem. Conventional therapy, however, reached the same treatment goal in less than 20% of the treated cases. Similarly, Becker et al (1988) and Caffesse et al (1990b) treated furcation defects using the guided tissue regeneration procedure and the Gore-Tex periodontal material. These authors reported results that were encouraging but not as good as those reported by Pontoriero et al (1988). An explanation for the difference could not be offered, apart from the possible impact of the plaque control program in which the patients were enrolled following surgical treatment. In the study by Pontoriero et al, during the 6-month healing period after surgical procedures, the patients were maintained on a plaque control program that included professional tooth cleaning and oral hygiene instruction once every 2 weeks. Nevertheless, both Becker et al and Caffesse et al concluded that guided tissue regeneration can improve the response to therapy of class II furcation defects. These results confirmed those of Gottlow et al (1986).

The use of guided tissue regeneration allows us to obtain significantly better results in the treatment of class II furcation and vertical osseous defects. More and more, therefore, this approach is being used in the treatment of severely advanced periodontal defects (Figs 7-10a to d).

## Studies using resorbable barriers

These reported studies have used a nonresorbable type of membrane that must be removed by a secondary surgical procedure. To make the clinical application of tooth isolation procedure practical, it is necessary to replace the nonresorbable barrier with a resorbable one. Recently, several investigators have shown that the gingival epithelium, as well as the gingival connective tissue, can be excluded from healing after periodontal surgery by the use of biodegradable barriers in dogs. Blumenthal et al (1986) used a purified bovine collagen gel over bone-grafted defects to inhibit epithelial migration into the defect. Magnusson et al (1988) reported on the use of a newly developed synthetic biodegradable material—polylactic acid membrane—during healing of surgical defects on premolars. Pitaru et al (1987, 1988, 1989) reported the effect of rat tail tendon collagen on the apical migration of epithelium during periodontal wound healing. They also reported partial regeneration of periodontal tissues following use of the collagen membranes. Card et al (1989) used Cargile (Ethicon, Somerville, NJ), a resorbable membrane derived from the cecum of an

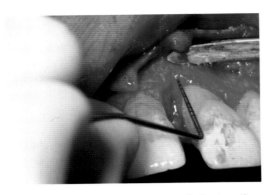

Fig 7-10a    Severe periodontal destruction around a maxillary central incisor. A 5-mm intrabony defect is present, with 12 mm of attachment loss.

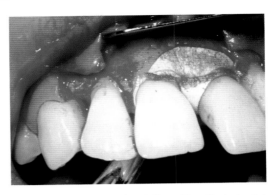

Fig 7-10b    Interproximal Gore-Tex Periodontal Material is adapted to the area after proper root instrumentation and debridement of the defect.

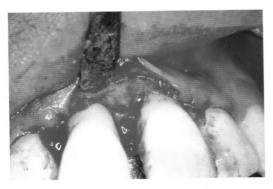

Fig 7-10c    Upon reentry, newly formed supporting tissues are seen. The distance from the cementoenamel junction to the alveolar crest is 4 mm throughout.

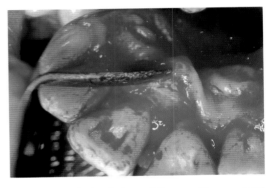

Fig 7-10d    Palatal view of the maxillary central incisor showing restoration of the interproximal bone in the area of the defect.

ox, to determine if a resorbable membrane that dissolved in a 30- to 60-day period would be an effective barrier in guided tissue regeneration procedures.

Nery et al (1990) determined whether the combination of porous biphasic calcium phosphate ceramic and fibrillar collagen gel, with and without citric acid root conditioning, would promote accelerated new attachment of periodontal tissue to the root surface in six dogs. Intrabony defects were surgically produced for each animal and were made

chronic for 16 weeks. These defects were assigned to two study treatment groups and one control group: ceramic-collagen with citric acid; ceramic-collagen without the acid; and surgical debridement and root planing only (control). The study demonstrated that the use of combined biphasic calcium phosphate ceramic and collagen is beneficial in promoting new attachment of periodontal tissues to the root surface. However, citric acid root conditioning does as well or better than ceramic-collagen alone.

In general, these studies using resorbable membranes demonstrated that gingival epithelium and connective tissue can be effectively diverted from the initial healing of root surfaces, thereby enhancing the formation of new attachment and bone. However, the problem that most investigators faced when dealing with the biodegradable membranes was the difficulty in handling the material. These collagen membranes were difficult to cut and position on the surgical site and were easily torn. They were prematurely resorbed in areas where inflammation could not be fully controlled (Card et al 1989).

A human study was performed to test the contribution of root conditioning and grafts to guided tissue regeneration in selected supracrestal/dehiscence defects, class II and III furcation defects, and wide intrabony defects (Schallhorn and McClain 1988). Ninety-five periodontal defects consisting of 62 furcation class II or III defects and 33 dehiscences, with horizontal bone loss or wide intrabony defects, were treated with Gore-Tex periodontal material. Seventy-five of these sites also received composite osseous grafting and citric acid root conditioning. All sites treated with either approach showed improvement in the clinical parameters (ie, probing depth reduction, gain in open and closed clinical attachment levels, and partial or complete furcation fill). The mean data for membrane alone and combined therapy demonstrated gains in open (reentry) vertical probing attachment levels of 4.5 to 5.3 mm, respectively, and gains in horizontal probing attachment levels of 3.1 to 4.2 mm, respectively, in furcations. No adverse clinical effects of the combined therapy were observed over use of membrane alone. Although block section removal was initially projected to evaluate the histologic response to therapy, no specimens were taken. Therefore, the microscopic effects of composite osseous grafting and citric acid root conditioning when used in conjunction with guided tissue regeneration membrane placement could not be assessed from this study.

Similarly, Garrett et al (1988) treated intraosseous periodontal defects with a combined adjunctive therapy of citric acid conditioning, bone grafting, and placement of collagenous membrane. A total of 25 proximal intraosseous defects were treated in 21 adult patients. The treatment included: (1) citric acid conditioning of the root surfaces; (2) grafting of particles of decalcified freeze-dried homologous bone, and (3) placement of freeze-dried homologous dura mater sheets between the replaced surgical flaps and the tooth surfaces. The results, as evaluated by probing attachment and probing bone level measurements, during 1 year of observation, demonstrated limited improvements of the treated defects. The limited results were similar to previous observations following treatment of intraosseous defects using different treatment modalities. New treatment approaches need to be sought to accomplish clinically significant and predictable regeneration in proximal intraosseous periodontal defects.

## Summary

Based on the review of a large number of studies on connective tissue regeneration, certain conclusions can be drawn:

1. New attachment is a biologic possibility, and the only method to verify such results is histologic analysis.
2. Because epithelial downgrowth along the root surface prevents new connective tissue attachment, it is imperative that apical migration of the epithelium be prevented to allow new attachment.
3. Whether or not a root was previously exposed to the oral environment seems of little importance in obtaining new attachment if the root has been properly prepared.

4. Cells derived from the periodontal ligament appear to be capable of promoting new connective tissue attachment.

5. At present, gingival connective tissue does not appear to be the source of progenitor cells for development of new attachment.

6. The formation of new connective tissue attachment is related to the possibility of guiding the growth of granulation tissue from source(s) that possess the biologic capacity of restoring the lost attachment apparatus.

7. The concept of controlling the cell repopulation in surgically treated areas is a logical extension of efforts to restore lost periodontium. Refinements in the published techniques and other innovative approaches will further enhance the clinician's ability to restore the periodontium.

# References

Albair WB, Cobb CM, Killoy WJ. Connective tissue attachment to periodontally diseased roots after citric acid demineralization. *J Periodontol* 1982;53: 515–526.

Aleo JJ, DeRenzis FA, Farber PA. In vitro attachment of human gingival fibroblasts to root surfaces. *J Periodontol* 1975;46:639–645.

Ali IU, Mautner V, Lanza R, Hynes RO. Restoration of normal morphology, adhesion and cytoskeleton in transformed cells by addition of transformed-sensitive surface protein. *Cell* 1977;11:115–126.

Andreasen JO, Hjorting-Hansen E. Replantation of teeth. II. Histological study of 22 replanted anterior teeth in humans. *Acta Odontol Scand* 1966;24: 287–306.

Andreasen JO. Histometric study of healing of periodontal tissues in rats after surgical injury. II. Healing events of alveolar bone, periodontal ligament and cementum. *Odontol Rev* 1976;27: 131–144.

Andreasen JO. Interrelation between alveolar bone and periodontal ligament repair after replantation of mature permanent incisors in monkeys. *J Periodont Res* 1981;16:228–235.

Andreasen JO, Kristerson L. The effect of limited drying or removal of the periodontal ligament. Periodontal healing after replantation of mature permanent incisors in monkeys. *Acta Odontol Scand* 1981;39:1–13.

Aukhil I, Pettersson E, Suggs C. Guided tissue regeneration. An experimental procedure in beagle dogs. *J Periodontol* 1986a;57:727–734.

Aukhil I, Simpson DM, Suggs C, Pettersson E. In vivo differentiation of progenitor cells of the periodontal ligament. *J Clin Periodontol* 1986b;13:862–868.

Aukhil I, Greco G, Suggs C, Torney D. Root resorption potential of granulation tissue from bone and flap connective tissue. *J Periodont Res* 1986c; 21:531–542.

Baker P, Evans R, Coburn R, Genco RJ. Tetracycline and its derivatives strongly bind to and are released from the tooth surface in active form. *J Periodontol* 1983;54:580–585.

Becker W, Becker BE, Berg L, Prichard J, Caffesse RG, Rosenberg E. New attachment after treatment with root isolation procedures: report for treated class III and class II furcations and vertical osseous defects. *Int J Periodont Res Dent* 1988; 8(3):9–23.

Bitterman PB, Rennard SI, Adelberg S, Crystal RG. Role of fibronectin as a growth factor for fibroblasts. *J Cell Biol* 1983;97:1925–1932.

Björn H. Experimental studies on reattachment. *Dent Pract* 1961;11:351–354.

Björn H, Hollender L, Lindhe J. Tissue regeneration in patients with periodontal disease. *Odontol Rev* 1965;16:317–326.

Bjorvatn K, Skaug N, Selvig KA. Inhibition of bacterial growth by tetracycline-impregnated enamel and dentin. *Scand J Dent Res* 1984;92:508–516.

Blumenthal NM, Sabet TW, Barrington E. Healing response to grafting of combined collagen-decalcified bone in periodontal wound healing. *J Periodontol* 1986;57:84–90.

Bogle G, Claffey N, Egelberg J. Healing of horizontal circumferential defects following regenerative surgery in beagle dogs. *J Clin Periodontol* 1985; 12:837–849.

Boyko GA, Melcher AH, Brunette DM. Formation of new periodontal ligament by periodontal ligament cells implanted in vivo after culture in vitro. *J Periodont Res* 1981;16:73–88.

Bowen JA, Mellonig JT, Gray JL, Towle HT. Comparison of decalcified freeze-dried bone allograft and porous particulate hydroxyapatite in human periodontal osseous defects. *J Periodontol* 1989; 60:647–654.

Bowers GM, Vargo JW, Levy B, Emerson JR, Bergquist JJ. Histologic observations following the placement of tricalcium phosphate implants in human intrabony defects. *J Periodontol* 1986;57: 286–287.

Bowers, GM, Chadroff B, Carnevale R, et al. Histologic evaluation of new attachment apparatus formation in humans. Part II. *J Periodontol* 1989a; 60:675–682.

Bowers, GM, Chadroff B, Carnevale R, et al. Histologic evaluation of new attachment apparatus formation in humans. Part III. *J Periodontol* 1989b; 60:683–693.

Caffesse RG, Holden MJ, Kon S, Nasjleti CE. The effect of citric acid and fibronectin application on healing following surgical treatment of naturally occurring periodontal disease in beagle dogs. *J Clin Periodontol* 1985;12:578–590.

Caffesse RG, Smith BS, Nasjleti CE, Lopatin DE. Cell proliferation after flap surgery, root conditioning and fibronectin application. *J Periodontol* 1987;58:661–666.

Caffesse RG, Kerry GJ, Chaves ES, et al. Clinical evaluation of the use of citric acid and autologous fibronectin in periodontal surgery. *J Periodontol* 1988a;59:565–569.

Caffesse RG, Smith BA, Castelli WA, Nasjleti CE. New attachment achieved by guided tissue regeneration in beagle dogs. *J Periodontol* 1988b;59:589–594.

Caffesse RG, Morrison EC, Kerry GJ, et al. Citric acid and autologous fibronectin in periodontal therapy. *J Dent Res* 1990a;69:276 (abstr 1338).

Caffesse RG, Smith BA, Duff B, Morrison EC, Merrill D, Becker W. Class II furcations treated by guided tissue regeneration in humans: case reports. *J Periodontol* 1990b;61:510–514.

Caffesse RG, Dominguez LE, Nasjleti CE, Castelli WA, Morrison EC, Smith BA. Furcation defects in dogs treated by guided tissue regeneration (GTR). *J Periodontol* 1990c;61:45–50.

Card SJ, Caffesse RG, Smith BA, Nasjleti CE. New attachment following the use of a resorbable membrane in the treatment of periodontitis in dogs. *Int J Periodont Rest Dent* 1989;9(1):59–69.

Caton J, Nyman S, Zander H. Histometric evaluation of periodontal surgery. II. Connective tissue attachment levels after four regenerative procedures. *J Clin Periodontol* 1980;7:224–231.

Claffey N, Bogle G, Bjorvatn K, Selvig KA, Egelberg J. Topical application of tetracycline in regenerative periodontal surgery in beagles. *Acta Odontol Scand* 1987;45:141–146.

Cole RT, Crigger M, Bogle G, Egelberg J, Selvig KA. Connective tissue regeneration to periodontally diseased teeth. A histological study. *J Periodont Res* 1980;15:1–9.

Dragoo MR. *Regeneration of the Periodontal Attachment in Humans.* Philadelphia: Lea & Febiger; 1981:95–101.

Egelberg J. Regeneration and repair of periodontal tissues. *J Periodont Res* 1987;22:233–242.

Ellegaard B, Karring T, Löe H. New periodontal attachment procedure based on retardation of epithelial migration. *J Clin Periodontol* 1974;1:75–88.

Ellegaard B, Nielsen IM, Karring T. Composite jaw and iliac cancellous bone grafts in intrabony defects in monkeys. *J Periodont Res* 1976a;11:299–310.

Ellegaard B, Karring T, Löe H. Retardation of epithelial migration in new attachment attempts in intrabony defects in monkeys. *J Clin Periodontol* 1976b;3:23–27.

Ericsson I, Lindhe J, Liljenberg B, Persson A. Lack of bacterial invasion in experimental periodontitis. *J Clin Periodontol* 1987;14:478–485.

Fernyhough W, Page RC. Attachment, growth and synthesis by human gingival fibroblasts on demineralized or fibronectin-treated normal and diseased tooth roots. *J Periodontol* 1983;54:133–140.

Frantz B, Polson A. Tissue interactions with dentin specimens after demineralization using tetracycline. *J Periodontol* 1988;59:714–721.

Froum SJ, Ortiz M, Witkin RT, Thaler R, Scopp IW, Stahl SS. Osseous autographs. III. Comparison of osseous coagulum-bone blend implants with open curettage. *J Periodontol* 1976;47:287–294.

Froum SJ, Kushner L, Scopp I, Stahl SS. Human clinical and histological responses to durapatite implants in intraosseous lesions. Case reports. *J Periodontol* 1982;54:719–725.

Gantes B, Martin M, Garrett S, Egelberg J. Treatment of periodontal furcation defects (II). Bone regeneration in mandibular class II defects. *J Clin Periodontol* 1988;15:232–239.

Gara GG, Adams DF. Implant therapy in human intrabony pockets: a review of the literature. *J Western Soc Periodontol/Periodont Abstr* 1981;29:32–47.

Garrett S, Loos B, Chamberlain D, Egelberg J. Treatment of intraosseous periodontal defects with a combined adjunctive therapy of citric acid conditioning, bone grafting and placement of collagenous membranes. *J Clin Periodontol* 1988;15:383–389.

Goldman I. A rationale for the treatment of the intrabony pocket: one method of treatment, subgingival curettage. *J Periodontol* 1949;20:83–91.

Golub LM, Wolff M, Lee HM, et al. Further evidence that tetracyclines inhibit collagenase activity in human crevicular fluid and from other mammalian sources. *J Periodontol* 1985;20:12–23.

Gottlow J, Nyman S, Karring T, Lindhe J. New attachment formation as a result of controlled tissue regeneration. *J Clin Periodontol* 1984;11:494–503.

Gottlow J, Nyman S, Lindhe J, Karring T, Wennstrom J. New attachment formation in the human periodontium by guided tissue regeneration. Case reports. *J Clin Periodontol* 1986;13:604–616.

Grinnell F, Bennett MH. Fibroblast adhesion on collagen substrata in the presence and absence of plasma fibronectin. *J Cell Sci* 1981;48:19–32.

Heaney T. Inhibition of fibroblast attachment. *J Clin Periodontol* 1986;13:987–994.

Hiatt WH, Schallhorn RG. Intraoral transplants of cancellous bone and marrow in periodontal lesions. *J Periodontol* 1973;44:194–208.

Isidor F, Karring T, Nyman S, Lindhe J. New attachment-reattachment following reconstructive periodontal surgery. *J Clin Periodontol* 1984;12:728–735.

Kalkwarf KL. Periodontal new attachment without the placement of osseous potentiating grafts. *Periodont Abstr* 1974;22:53–62.

Karring T, Nyman S, Lindhe J. Healing following implantation of periodontitis affected roots into bone tissue. *J Clin Periodontol* 1980;7:96–105.

Kenney EB, Lekovic V, Sa Ferreira JC, Han T, Dimitrijevic B, Carranza FA. Bone formation within porous hydroxylapatite implants in human periodontal defects. *J Periodontol* 1986;57:76–83.

Kleinman H, Klebe R, Martin G. Role of collagenous matrices in the adhesion and growth of cells. *J Cell Biol* 1981;88:473–485.

Klinge B, Nilveus R, Kiger RD, Egelberg J. Effect of flap placement and defect size on healing of experimental furcation defects. *J Periodont Res* 1981;16:236–248.

Klinge B, Nilveus R, Egelberg J. Effect of crown-attached sutures on healing of experimental furcation defects in dogs. *J Clin Periodontol* 1985; 12:369–373.

Knowles JW, Burgett FG, Nissle RR, Shick RA, Morrison EC, Ramfjord SP. Results of periodontal treatment related to pocket depth and attachment level. Eight years. *J Periodontol* 1979;50:225–233.

Kurkinen M, Vaheri A, Roberts PJ, Stenman S. Sequential appearance of fibronectin and collagen in experimental granulation tissue. *Lab Invest* 1980; 43:47–51.

Line SE, Polson AM, Zander HA. Relationship between periodontal injury, selective cell repopulation and ankylosis. *J Periodontol* 1974;45:725–730.

Listgarten MA, Rosenberg MM. Histological study of repair following new attachment procedures in human periodontal lesions. *J Periodontol* 1979;50: 333–344.

Löe H, Waerhaug J. Experimental replantation of teeth in dogs and monkeys. *Arch Oral Biol* 1961; 3:176–184.

Lynch SE, Nixon JN, Colvin RB, Antoniades HN. Role of platelet-derived growth factor in wound healing: synergistic effects with other growth factors. *Proc Natl Acad Sci USA* 1987;84:7696–7700.

Lynch SE, Williams RC, Polson AM, et al. A combination of platelet-derived and insulin-like growth factors enhances periodontal regeneration. *J Clin Periodontol* 1989;16:545–548.

Magnusson I, Claffey N, Bogle G, Garrett S, Egelberg J. Root resorption following periodontal flap procedures in monkeys. *J Periodont Res* 1985a;20: 79–85.

Magnusson I, Nyman S, Karring T, Egelberg J. Connective tissue attachment formation following exclusion of gingival connective tissue and epithelium during healing. *J Periodont Res* 1985b;20: 201–208.

Magnusson I, Batich C, Collins BR. New attachment formation following controlled tissue regeneration using biodegradable membranes. *J Periodontol* 1988;59:1–6.

Martin M, Gantes B, Garrett S, Egelberg J. Treatment of periodontal furcation defects (I). Review of the literature and description of a regenerative surgical technique. *J Clin Periodontol* 1988;15:227–231.

McCulloch CAG, Nemeth E, Lowenberg B, Melcher AH. Paravascular cells in endosteal spaces of alveolar bone contribute to periodontal ligament cell populations. *Anat Record* 1987;219:233–242.

McHugh WD. The effects of exclusion of epithelium from healing periodontal pockets. *J Periodontol* 1988;59:750–757.

Meffert RM, Thomas JR, Hamilton KM, Brownstein CN. Hydroxylapatite as an alloplastic graft in the treatment of human periodontal osseous defects. *J Periodontol* 1985;56:63–73.

Melcher AH. Repair of wounds in the periodontium of the rat. Influence of periodontal ligament on osteogenesis. *Arch Oral Biol* 1970;15:1183–1204.

Melcher AH. On the repair potential of periodontal tissues. *J Periodontol* 1976;47:256–260.

Melcher AH, Cheong T, Cox J, Nemeth E, Shiga A. Synthesis of cementum-like tissue in vitro by cells cultured from bone: a light and electron microscope study. *J Periodont Res* 1986;21:592–612.

Mellonig JT. Decalcified freeze-dried bone allograft as an implant material in human periodontal defects. *Int J Periodont Rest Dent* 1984;4(4):41–55.

Moskow BS, Karsh F, Stein SD. Histological assessment of autogenous bone graft: a case report and critical evaluation. *J Periodontol* 1979;50:291–300.

Nasjleti CE, Castelli WA, Blankenship JR. The storage of teeth before reimplantation in monkeys. *Oral Surg* 1975a;39:20–29.

Nasjleti CE, Caffesse RG, Castelli WA, Hoke JA. Healing after tooth reimplantation in monkeys. A radioautographic study. *Oral Surg* 1975b;39: 361–375.

Nasjleti CE, Caffesse RG, Castelli WA, Lopatin DE, Kowalski CJ. Effect of lyophilized autologous plasma on periodontal healing of replanted teeth. *J Periodontol* 1986;57:568–578.

Nasjleti CE, Caffesse RG, Castelli WA, Lopatin DE, Kowalski CJ. Effect of fibronectin on healing of replanted teeth in monkeys: a histologic and autoradiographic study. *Oral Surg Oral Med Oral Pathol* 1987;63:291–299.

Nery EB, Eslami A, Van Swol RL. Biphasic calcium phosphate ceramic combined with fibrillar collagen with and without citric acid conditioning in the treatment of periodontal osseous defects. *J Periodontol* 1990;61:166–172.

Nilveus R, Bogle G, Crigger M, Egelberg J, Selvig K. The effect of topical citric acid application on the healing of experimental furcation defects in dogs. II. Healing after repeated surgery. *J Periodontol Res* 1980;15:544–550.

Nojima N, Koyabashi M, Shionome M, Takahashi N, Suda T, Hasegawa K. Fibroblastic cells derived from bovine periodontal ligaments have the phenotypes of osteoblasts. *J Periodont Res* 1990;25:179–185.

Nyman S, Karring T, Lindhe J, Planten S. Healing following implantation of periodontitis-affected roots into gingival connective tissue. *J Clin Periodontol* 1980;7:394–401.

Nyman S, Gottlow J, Karring T, Lindhe J. The regenerative potential of the periodontal ligament. An experimental study in the monkey. *J Clin Periodontol* 1982a;9:257–265.

Nyman S, Lindhe J, Karring T, Rylander H. New attachment following surgical treatment of human periodontal disease. *J Clin Periodontol* 1982b;9:290–296.

Pearlstein E. Plasma membrane glycoprotein which mediates adhesion of fibroblasts to collagen. *Nature* 1976;262:497–500.

Peltzman B, Bowers GM, Reddi AH, Bergquist JJ. Treatment of furcation involvements with fibronectin and intraoral autogenous bone grafts: preliminary observations. *Int J Periodont Rest Dent* 1988;8(5):51–63.

Pettersson EC, Aukhil I. Citric acid conditioning of roots affects guided tissue regeneration in experimental periodontal wounds. *J Periodont Res* 1986;21:543–552.

Pitaru S, Tal H, Soldinger M, Grosskopf A, Noff N. Collagen membranes prevent the apical migration of epithelium during periodontal wound healing. *J Periodont Res* 1987;22:331–333.

Pitaru S, Tal H, Soldinger M, Grosskopf A, Noff M. Partial regeneration of periodontal tissues using collagen barriers. Initial observations in the canine. *J Periodontol* 1988;59:380–386.

Pitaru S, Tal H, Soldinger M, Noff M. Collagen membranes prevent apical migration of epithelium and support new connective tissue attachment during periodontal wound healing in dogs. *J Periodont Res* 1989;24:247–253.

Polson AM, Caton J. Factors influencing periodontal repair and regeneration. *J Periodontol* 1982;53:617–625.

Pommier CG, Inada S, Fries LF, Takahashi T, Frank MM, Brown EJ. Plasma fibronectin enhances phagocytosis of opsonized particles of human peripheral blood monocytes. *J Exp Med* 1983;157:1844–1854.

Pontoriero R, Lindhe J, Nyman S, Karring T, Rosenberg E, Sanavi F. Guided tissue regeneration in degree II furcation-involved mandibular molars. A clinical study. *J Clin Periodontol* 1988;15:247–254.

Proye MP, Polson AM. The effect of root surface alterations on periodontal healing. I. Surgical denudation. *J Clin Periodontol* 1982a;9:428–440.

Proye MP, Polson AM. Repair in different zones of the periodontium after tooth reimplantation. *J Periodontol* 1982b;53:379–389.

Ramfjord SP, Nissle RR. The modified Widman flap. *J Periodontol* 1974;45:601–607.

Ramfjord SP, Knowles JW, Nissle RR, Burgett FG, Shick RA. Results following three modalities of periodontal therapy. *J Periodontol* 1975;46:522–526.

Register AA, Burdick FA. Accelerated reattachment with cementogenesis to dentin, demineralized in situ. II. Defect repair. *J Periodontol* 1976;47:497–505.

Renvert S, Egelberg J. Healing after treatment of periodontal intraosseous defects. III. Effects of osseous grafting and citric acid conditioning. *J Clin Periodontol* 1981;12:441–455.

Renvert S, Garrett S, Shallhorn RG, Egelberg J. Healing after treatment of periodontal intraosseous defects. III. Effect of osseous grafting and citric acid conditioning. *J Clin Periodontol* 1985;12:441–455.

Rosling B, Nyman S, Lindhe J, Jern B. The healing potential of the periodontal tissues following different techniques of periodontal surgery in plaque-free dentitions. A 2-year clinical study. *J Clin Periodontol* 1976;3:233–250.

Rummelhart JM, Mellonig JT, Gray JL, Towle HJ. Comparison of freeze-dried bone allograft and demineralized freeze-dried bone allograft in human periodontal osseous defects. *J Periodontol* 1989;60:655–663.

Ruoslahti E, Vaheri A. Interaction of soluble fibroblast surface antigen with fibrinogen and fibrin. Identity with cold insoluble globulin of human plasma. *J Exp Med* 1975;141:497–501.

Schallhorn RG, McClain PK. Combined osseous composite grafting, root conditioning, and guided tissue regeneration. *Int J Periodont Rest Dent* 1988;8(4):9–31.

Smith BA, Mason WE, Morrison EC, Caffesse RG. The effectiveness of citric acid as an adjunct to surgical re-attachment procedures in humans. *J Clin Periodontol* 1986;13:701–708.

Smith BA, Caffesse RG, Nasjleti CE, Kon S, Castelli WA. Effects of citric acid and fibronectin and laminin application in treating periodontitis. *J Clin Periodontol* 1987a;14:396–402.

Smith BA, Smith JS, Caffesse RG, Nasjleti CE, Lopatin DE, Kowalski CJ. Effect of citric acid and various concentrations of fibronectin on healing following periodontal flap surgery in dogs. *J Periodontol* 1987b;58:667–673.

Somerman MJ, Foster RA, Vorsteg GM, Progebin K, Wynn RL. Effects of minocycline on fibroblast attachment and spreading. *J Periodont Res* 1988;23:154–159.

Stahl SS, Froum SJ. Human clinical and histologic repair responses following the use of citric acid in periodontal therapy. *J Periodontol* 1977;48:261–266.

Steiner SR, Crigger M, Egelberg J. Connective tissue regeneration to periodontally diseased teeth. II. Histologic observations. *J Periodont Res* 1981;16:109–116.

Tanner MG, Solt CW, Vuddhakanok S. An evaluation of new attachment formation using a microfibrillar collagen barrier. *J Periodontol* 1988;59:524–530.

Terranova VP, Martin GR. Molecular factors determining gingival tissue interaction with tooth structure. *J Periodont Res* 1982;17:530–533.

Terranova VP, Franzetti LC, Hic S, et al. A biochemical approach to periodontal regeneration: Tetracycline treatment of dentin promotes fibroblast adhesion and growth. *J Periodont Res* 1986;21:330–337.

Terranova VP, Wikesjö UME. Extracellular matrices and polypeptide growth factors as mediators of functions of cells of the periodontium. A review. *J Periodontol* 1987;58:371–380.

Terranova VP, Hic S, Franzetti L, Lyall RM, Wikesjö UME. A biochemical approach to periodontal regeneration. AFSCM: Assay for specific cell migration. *J Periodontol* 1987;58:247–257.

Terranova VP, Odziemiec C, Tweden KS, Spadone DP. Repopulation of dentin surfaces by periodontal ligament cells and endothelial cells: effect of basic fibroblast growth factor. *J Periodontol* 1989; 60:293–301.

Walker C, Pappas J, Tyler K, Cohen S, Gordon J. Antibiotic susceptibilities of periodontal bacteria: in vitro susceptibilities to eight antimicrobial agents. *J Periodontol* 1985;56(Suppl):67–74.

Weiss R, Reddi AH. Role of fibronectin in collagenous matrix induced mesenchymal cell proliferation and differentiation in vivo. *Exp Cell Res* 1981;133: 247–254.

Wikesjö UME, Baker PJ, Christersson LA, et al. A biochemical approach to periodontal regeneration. Tetracycline treatment conditions dentin surfaces. *J Periodont Res* 1986;21:322–329.

Wikesjö UME, Claffey N, Christersson LA, et al. Repair of periodontal furcation defects in beagle dogs following reconstructive surgery including root surface demineralization with tetracycline hydrochloride and topical fibronectin application. *J Clin Periodontol* 1988;15:73–80.

Wirthlin MR. Growth substances: potential use in periodontics. *J Western Soc Periodontol/Periodont Abstr* 1989;37:101–126.

Yamada KM, Weston JA. Isolation of major cell surface glycoprotein from fibroblasts. *Proc Natl Acad Sci* [USA] 1974;71:3492–3496.

Yamada KM, Olden K, Pastan I. Transformation sensitive cell surface protein: isolation, characterization, and role in cellular morphology and adhesion. *Ann NY Acad Sci* 1978;312:256–277.

Yamada KM, Akiyama SK, Hasegawa T, et al. Recent advances in research on fibronectin and other cell attachment proteins. *J Cell Biochem* 1985;28: 79–97.

Yukna RA, Mayer ET, Brite DV. Longitudinal evaluation of durapatite ceramic as an alloplastic implant in periodontal osseous defects after 3 years. *J Periodontol* 1984;55:633–637.

Zamet JS. A comparative clinical study of three periodontal surgical techniques. *J Clin Periodontol* 1975;2:87–97.

# Chapter 8

# Guided Tissue Regeneration for Periodontal Defects

William Becker

The main goal of periodontal therapy is the restoration of the periodontium that has been destroyed by periodontal diseases. Restitution of the periodontium has often been an elusive, frustrating objective of therapy. According to Hancock (1989), procedures that may generate new attachment are flap debridement, bone grafting, and guided tissue regeneration. The American Academy of Periodontology (1986) defines *new attachment:* "The reunion of connective tissue with a root surface that has been deprived of its periodontal ligament. This reunion occurs by the formation of new cementum with inserting fibers."

This chapter will discuss flap debridement and guided tissue regeneration as methods for attaining new attachment. (Bone grafting procedures are discussed in chapter 5.)

## Defect anatomy

An understanding of osseous defect anatomy is important in diagnosing periodontal defects that may respond to new attachment procedures. An intrabony defect re-sults when the junctional epithelium is apical to the alveolar crest. Goldman and Cohen (1958) classified intrabony defects according to the number of bony walls surrounding the defects. Several authors have reported on the incidence and location of intrabony defects (Lorato 1974; Monson and Nichollson 1974; Saari et al 1968; Tal 1984). Intrabony defects are frequently found in areas of the mouth where the cortical bone is thick and is separated by a large volume of cancellous bone. Saari et al (1968) reported that the most common location of intrabony defects is the mesial interproximal location between the maxillary and mandibular second molars. As inflammation spreads apically, cancellous bone is resorbed, leaving various types of osseous abberations. Because the mandible widens anteroposteriorly, the incidence of intrabony defects increases in the posterior regions of the mandible. Funnel-shaped defects are frequently found in the maxilla; however, these defects are not as deep as those found in the mandible.

When furcations are treated with new attachment procedures, root trunk length, interradicular loss of attachment, root proximity, buccolingual attachment loss, and depth of a vertical component are important diagnostic anatomic factors. Tal and Lemmer (1982) reported a high incidence of furcation involvements on the buccal aspects of mandibular first molars. As the depth of the furcation invasion deepens, the height of the alveolar crest tends to decrease. The mandibular second molar frequently has a combination vertical defect and horizontal furcation involvement.

The enlightened clinician bases treatment of bony defects on an understanding of anatomy, defect location, and limitations for each procedure. Preoperative patient records should consist of accurate clinical probing depths and attachment levels and good-quality radiographs. Although these records are essential to making a diagnosis and treatment plan, the final treatment plan for specific defects is made with accurate radiographs and after flap reflection and defect debridement.

# Flap debridement and interproximal denudation

Over the past 30 years there have been many reports on the successful treatment of intrabony defects (Becker et al 1986a, 1986b; Carranza 1954; Ellegaard et al 1974, 1976; Froum et al 1982; Goldman 1949; Polson and Heijl 1978; Prichard 1957a, 1957b, 1960, 1983; Renvert et al 1981; Rosling et al 1976). In most instances, the defects were accessed after surgical flap reflection. Most reports indicate that the greatest amount of bone fill occurs in combination two- and three-walled defects and three-walled intrabony defects. One-walled or hemiseptal defects usually have the least amount of bone fill.

In 1957, Prichard presented clinical documentation of successfully treated three-wall intrabony defects. The three-wall defect was carefully defined as having three bony walls adjacent to the tooth surface with the root forming the fourth wall. The defects treated by Prichard did not involve furcations and had definite bony stops. Prichard (1957a) excised the gingival margin from the flaps and thoroughly debrided the defects. Calculus was removed from the root surfaces, but deliberate removal of all root cementum was not attempted. By excising the gingival flap margin, Prichard felt that epithelium was delayed from reaching the root surface, thereby allowing time for clot organization. The clinical documentation as demonstrated by radiographic changes and reentry procedures clearly showed significant amounts of bone fill in very extensive bony defects. Teeth treated this way have been maintained for more than 30 years.

Polson and Heijl (1978) treated two- and three-walled intrabony defects with open flap curettage. After thorough defect and root instrumentation, maximum flap coaptation was achieved. Results from this study indicated postoperative decreases in probing depth and gains in clinical attachment levels. These changes were substantiated by reentry procedures. There was an average increase of 2.5 mm in bone levels with minimal crestal resorption. Becker et al (1986a, 1986b) treated three-walled intrabony defects by flap curettage procedures. In the majority of treated sites the flaps covered the defects. Results from this study indicated a 2.7-mm mean gain in clinical attachment level and an average of 2.5-mm of gain in bone level. Volumetric analysis of defects indicated a 50% decrease in defect volume for half of the defects treated. There were no apparent differences in clinical results between wide-, medium-, and narrow-mouthed defects. The results from most studies evaluating treatment of two- and three-walled intrabony defects have indicated that after flap curettage, deep three-walled intrabony defects appear to have the greatest amount of bone fill. Two-walled intrabony defects can be treated by this method; however, the results do not seem to be as predictable as for the three-walled intrabony defect.

New attachment can be accurately measured and evaluated clinically, but, according to Gara and Adams (1981), absolute proof of new attachment can only be demonstrated from histologic sections. During surgery, calculus on the root surface should be notched. New attachment as a result of surgical therapy can be measured from fixed grooves in the root surface. Although histologic evaluation provides the most convincing evidence of new attachment, it is difficult to retrieve successfully treated teeth for histologic study. From animal and limited human biopsy specimens of intrabony defects treated by debridement, it appears that healing occurs by new bone formation and a long junctional epithelium (Caton et al 1980; Stahl et al 1982).

## Surgical treatment for intrabony defects

Defects that may be candidates for treatment by flap curettage are usually not heavily instrumented prior to surgery. On a purely empirical level, many clinicians think an inflamed lesion may respond to therapy more favorably than one that has been heavily instrumented prior to surgery. The rationale for this approach is that marrow spaces may be open and immature collagen may be present in the inflamed lesion. The tissue factors in the inflamed lesion may be more responsive to rapid healing than are those found in the chronic lesion. This hypothesis has yet to be tested (Becker 1986a; Prichard 1957a).

Access for treatment of intrabony defects is made by reflecting full-thickness buccolingual mucoperiosteal flaps. Adequate flap reflection is a prerequisite for proper defect visibility and instrumentation. Poorly designed flaps often result in surgical trauma to the tissues. The granulation tissue is best removed with curets and rotary instruments. After the granulation tissue has been completely removed, the roots are instrumented with a combination of ultrasonic scalers, fine rotary instruments, files, and small curets. These instruments are also used to meticulously debride the osseous defect. After a thorough debridement, the roots and defect are examined to determine defect depth and number of osseous walls. If the majority of the defect is surrounded by three deep bony walls, it is irrigated with water or sterile saline and sutured for maximum flap closure. The use of dressing is optional, and its use does not appear to affect proper healing. If dressings are not applied, patients can begin gentle brushing along the flap-tooth junction on the second postoperative day. Antimicrobial agents can be applied at the discretion of the surgeon. Sutures are removed in 7 days.

Rosling et al (1976) have demonstrated the importance of thorough plaque removal postsurgery. Patients with low plaque scores have the greatest decreases in probing depth, gains in clinical attachment levels, and increases in bone levels. Patients with poor oral hygiene have minimal changes in clinical measurements. Although intrabony defects treated by flap curettage have produced successful long-term results, this procedure may not produce new attachment.

## Biologic principles relating to new attachment

Melcher (1976) presented the biologic principles that have become the basis for subsequent studies relating to new attachment procedures. He divided the periodontium into four compartments: gingival epithelium, gingival connective tissue, bone, and periodontal membrane. The periodontal membrane was considered the primary source of cells necessary for periodontal regeneration. The endosteum of bone was also considered to be a source of undifferentiated cells. These cells may also play an important role in the regenerative process.

In the late 1970s and 1980s, a series of studies was undertaken to determine the origin of cells necessary for new attachment (Aukhil et al 1983; Caton et al 1980; Isidor et al 1988; Karring et al 1980, 1983; Nyman et al 1980, 1982a, 1982b). Caton et al (1980) induced experimental periodontitis in monkeys. Four treatments were evaluated in terms of their ability to form new attachment on periodontitis-affected roots: scaling and root planing, modified Widman flap surgery, defect and root debridement, and implantation of frozen red marrow and beta tricalcium phosphate. The results indicated that all procedures healed by formation of a long junctional epithelium with varying degrees of new bone formation.

Our insight into the origin of periodontal regenerative cells has been enlightened by a series of studies performed by the "Scandinavian group." The following is a brief summary of their studies. Karring et al (1980) devitalized periodontitis-affected roots and transplanted them into surgically created bony defects. The diseased portion of the root underwent resorption and ankylosis. The portion of the root with retained periodontal ligament showed evidence of reattachment to the root surface. In another study (Karring et al 1983), a similar experiment was performed but incisions were made over the roots, thereby allowing epithelium to proliferate along the connective tissue. When epithelium was present along the root surface, ankylosis

and root resorption did not occur. From this study it was hypothesized that epithelium may act as a protective barrier and thus prevent root resorption and ankylosis. Nyman and coworkers (1982a) created fenestration defects over the labial surfaces of monkey canines. They removed 2 to 3 mm of bone and periodontal ligament, thus creating a fenestration defect over the root. The cementum was removed from the root surface. Millipore filters (Bedford, MA) were placed over the defects to prevent gingival connective tissue from contacting the defects. Biopsy specimens of the experimental areas revealed new attachment consisting of new cementum with inserting fibers and restitution of the alveolar bone. The conclusions from this study indicated that the periodontal membrane may be a very important source of progenitor cells if new attachment is to occur.

It appears that the periodontal membrane is an important source of cells necessary for new attachment; however, other tissue compartments may also play an important role in the regenerative process. Studies by Iglhaut et al (1988) indicated that alveolar bone may also play a significant role in the regenerative process. Recently, Melcher et al (1986) have presented results from an in vitro study that suggested the progeny of bone cells may be able to produce cementumlike substances. The influence of bone in the regenerative process may be dependent on the influences of the local environment. Results from the above studies present strong evidence for the importance of the periodontal membrane and endosteum in the regenerative process.

Nyman et al (1982) demonstrated the clinical reality of gaining new attachment on a periodontitis-affected root. The biologic rationale for their clinical trial was based on the biologic principles learned from the previously cited studies. They treated a patient with a severely involved mandibular incisor. After flap reflection, a notch was placed at the level of the alveolar crest. Meticulous defect and root surface debridement were performed. A Millipore filter was placed over the defect and luted to the crown. The flaps were replaced, and after 3 months a block section of the treated site was removed and histologically evaluated. New cementum with inserting fibers were present 5 mm coronal to the notch in the alveolar crest. Varying amounts of bone formation were seen in the shallow intrabony defect. This study indicated that if gingival epithelium and connective tissue are excluded from the healing process, new attachment can occur. Cell repopulation of the previously diseased root surface presumably came from the periodontal ligament.

Gottlow et al (1984a) and Caffesse et al (1988) used the principles of guided tissue regeneration (GTR) to treat extensive defects in experimental animals. Gottlow and coworkers removed 50% to 75% of the alveolar bone from monkey teeth. Periodontitis was then allowed to develop. After 3 months the osseous defects were treated by flap debridement alone or with Millipore or polytetrafluoroethylene (PTFE) membrane placement and flap debridement. Membranes were placed supragingivally and glued to the clinical crowns. Biopsy specimens of the treated sites demonstrated that significant new attachment had occurred at the test sites. For test sites, the amount of new bone ranged from 20% to 100% of the exposed roots. The greatest amount of new attachment occurred at sites treated with PTFE membranes. In some instances cementum formed within the membranes.

## Materials used for guided tissue regeneration

The purpose of placing materials over osseous defects is to exclude gingival epithe-

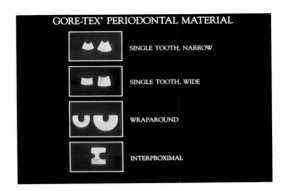

Fig 8-1 Various shapes of periodontal material. Appropriate shape is dictated by size, location, and defect being treated.

lium and connective tissue from the root surface. The space created by these materials allows cells from the periodontal membrane to populate the root surface. Ideally, these materials should be sterile, biocompatible, resorb slowly, create sufficient space for cell repopulation, and should be relatively easy to place surgically.

To date, Gore-Tex Periodontal Material (W.L. Gore and Associates, Flagstaff, Ariz) has been the most widely used material for GTR procedures. The popularity of this material is based on extensive laboratory and clinical trials. The material is made from polytetrafluoroethylene and consists of an open microstructure collar and an occlusive apron. The collar allows a space for clot formation and early collagen penetration. The clot and immature collagen fibrils may stop epithelial proliferation by contact inhibition (Winter 1974). Because the apron is occlusive, gingival epithelium and connective tissue cannot come into contact with the root surface; therefore, new attachment can only come for cells from the periodontal ligament or endosteum. The periodontal material is commercially available in various sizes and shapes to accommodate defect morphology and location (Fig 8-1). The material is provided in a sterile envelope, is biocompatible, and is nonresorbable.

Biodegradeable and collagen membranes have been successfully used to treat various types of bony defects in laboratory animals (Blumenthal et al 1988; Magnusson et al 1985, 1987; Pitaru et al 1987, 1988). Use of these materials has not been reported in human clinical trials. The potential value of collagen membranes is that they resorb and consequently do not require a second surgical procedure.

## Surgery for guided tissue regeneration and clinical results

The objective of GTR procedures is to gain new clinical attachment, improve bone levels, and minimize postoperative recession. Several clinical investigations have reported successful treatment of intrabony as well as furcation defects with GTR procedures (Becker et al 1987, 1988; Gottlow et al 1986; Pontoriero et al 1987, 1988; Schallhorn and McClain 1988). Gottlow et al (1986) presented an impressive number of clinical cases of treatment with flap curettage, root and defect instrumentation, and PTFE membrane placement. Human biopsy specimens showed histologic evidence of new attachment. Becker et al (1987) reentered several sites that were treated with GTR procedures. Partial-thickness dissections were used to gain access to the treated furcations. The new tissue was not bone but was firmly attached to the tooth and resisted probe penetration. The changes in probing depth were termed "open probing new attachment."

Becker et al (1988) subsequently reported clinical findings on vertical and furcation defects treated with GTR procedures. For vertical defects there was a mean decrease in probing depth of 6.4 mm, a gain in probing attachment of 4.5 mm, and a mean decrease in defect depth

of 4.5 mm. These changes have been sustained over a 5-year observation period. The clinical results for treated vertical and some class II furcation involvements by GTR procedures appear to be fairly predictable. Pontoriero et al (1987, 1988) reported results after treatment of class III and II furcation involvements, but, although the results are encouraging, most clinicians consider treatment of class III furcations by GTR procedures to be unpredictable.

Ideal defects for GTR procedures are three-walled defects, combination two- and three-walled defects, and funnel-shaped defects with definite osseous stops. The defects should be greater than 5 mm deep. Class II furcations with or without a vertical component can also be successfully treated.

Osseous defects chosen for GTR procedures are accessed by full-thickness buccolingual flaps. Efforts are made to retain the interdental papillae. To gain adequate access for proper defect debridement, vertical releasing incisions should be made two teeth anterior to the tooth being treated. To decrease the incidence of flap necrosis, use of relatively thick flaps is recommended. After flap reflection, defects are fastidiously debrided with hand curets and rotary instruments. Calculus deposits are thoroughly removed from root surfaces by a combination of ultrasonic, rotary, and hand instrumentation.

After the defect has been diagnosed as appropriate for a GTR procedure, an appropriately sized periodontal membrane is chosen. The material should completely cover and extend a minimum of 4 mm apical to the defect. The material should also extend 2 to 3 mm over the lateral borders of the entire defect. The collar of the material should be at or slightly below the cementoenamel junction. The material is tightly secured to the tooth by a sling suture. Interrupted interdental sutures are then used to adapt the flaps. The vertical

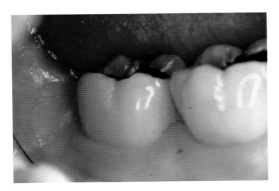

Fig 8-2a    Preoperative view.

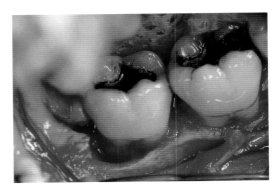

Fig 8-2b    Defect involves the distal and facial aspects of the tooth. There is a class II furcation involvement from the buccal aspect. Note calculus on distal line angle.

incisions are sutured after complete coverage of the material has been achieved.

Becker et al (1989) have proposed a variation of this suturing method. When the contact relationship of adjacent teeth are tight, the suture is passed through the buccal flap and over the contact area. The suture is then passed through the lingual flap and back over the contact to the buccal tooth aspect. The flaps are moved coronally by placing slight tension on the suture. Once the flaps are located on the clinical crown, the suture can be firmly secured with a knot. This suturing method allows flap placement onto the clinical crown and is based on a similar technique described by Gantes et al (1988). The purpose of coronal flap placement is to increase the distance the epithelium must migrate before it reaches the membrane collar. Increasing the distance necessary for epithelial migration may allow clot organization within the membrane collar.

Patients receive tetracycline hydrochloride or other compounds containing tetracycline (250 mg, qid, for 1 week) and instructed to begin gentle brushing at the flap margin on the second postoperative day. If interdental sutures were used, they should not be removed until the third or fourth postoperative week. If the sutures are placed over the contacts, they will loosen in about 14 days and will need to be removed. In this case, in about 4 to 6 weeks the flap margins will recede to or be slightly coronal to the cementoenamel junction.

Within 4 to 6 weeks after surgery it is necessary to remove the periodontal material. Infiltration anesthesia is administered and a scalpel is used to dissect the inner layer of the flap from the material. The knot securing the material is identified and released. The material can then be gently released from the inner border of the flap with the scalpel. The new granulation tissue lining the treated defect must not be disturbed. Once the material is removed, the inner border of the flap margins is thinned with a small diamond rotary instrument. The flap margins are sutured with either gut or silk sutures. The sutures are removed in a week and the patients are placed into a maintenance program.

Patients treated and maintained by GTR procedures are presented in Figs 8-2 through 8-4 and Table 8-1.

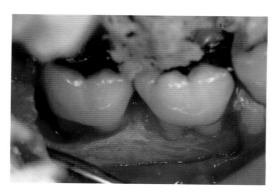

Fig 8-2c    Defect and root have been thoroughly debrided.

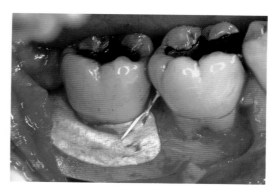

Fig 8-2d    Periodontal material has been adapted to defect and root surface by means of a PTFE suture.

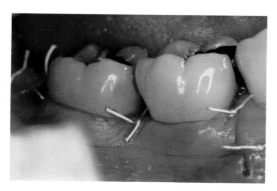

Fig 8-2e    The flaps have been sutured with PTFE interrupted sutures.

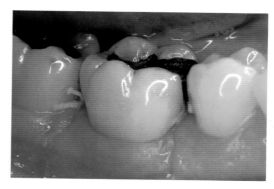

Fig 8-2f    View at 2-week postoperative visit. Sutures are still in place.

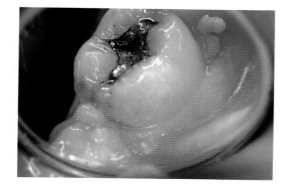

Fig 8-2g    View at 6-week postoperative visit. Material is completely covered. Material was removed at this visit.

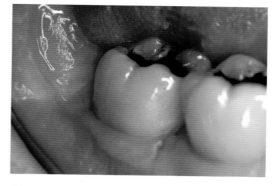

Fig 8-2h    View at 9-month recall visit. Gingival margin is at the cementoenamel junction. There was a 5-mm reduction in probing depth and a 4-mm gain in clinical attachment level.

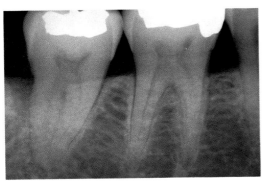 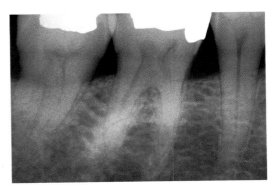

Figs 8-2i and j   Preoperative and 9-month radiographs. Closure of distal intrabony defect is visible. (Note: remount radiograph was used to show more of distal aspect.)

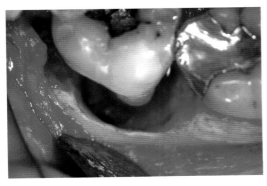 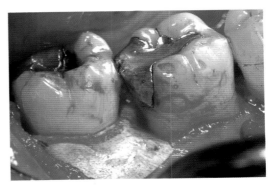

Fig 8-3a   The mandibular molar has a combination facial intraosseous defect and a class II furcation invasion. The vertical component of the defect extends to the mesial aspect of the tooth.

Fig 8-3b.   PTFE periodontal material has been sutured tightly around the defect.

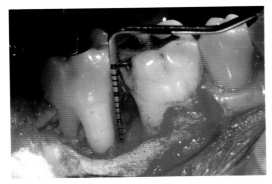 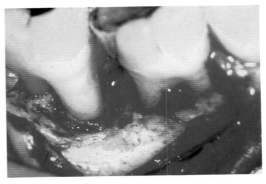

Fig. 8-3c   Nine-month reentry. There is an average increase in bone level of 5 mm. Defect is now an incipient class I involvement.

Fig 8-3d   The slight residual bony defect has been reduced with osseous contouring.

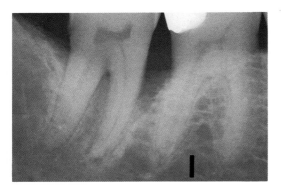

Fig 8-3e

Fig 8-3e to g   Initial, 9-month, and 2.5-year follow-up radiographs. Note improvement in furcation and interproximal osseous levels.

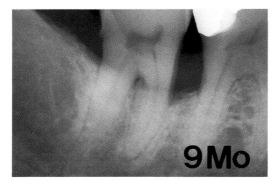

Fig 8-3f

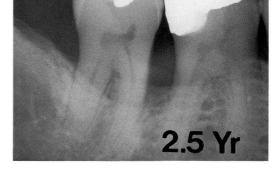

Fig 8-3g

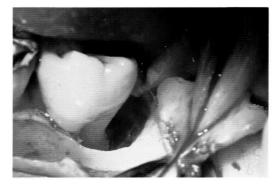

Fig 8-4a   Wide, three-walled intrabony defect. Buccal aspect.

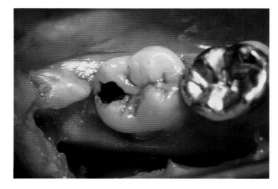

Fig 8-4b   Lingual view showing uninvolved furcation.

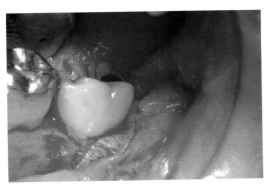

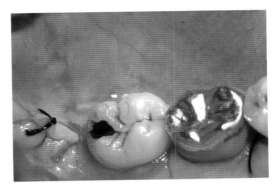

Fig 8-4c   Periodontal material has been sutured in place.

Fig 8-4d   Flaps have been sutured for maximum closure.

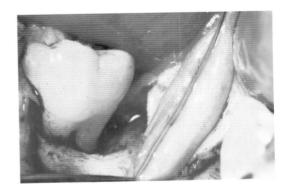

Fig 8-4e   Nine-month reentry. There are a 5.5-mm increase in bone level and a 1-mm residual osseous defect.

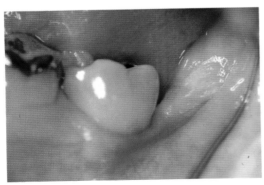

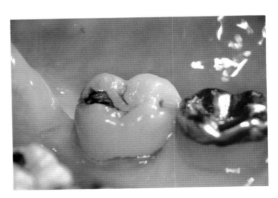

Fig 8-4f and g   Buccal and lingual views taken at 3-year maintenance visit.

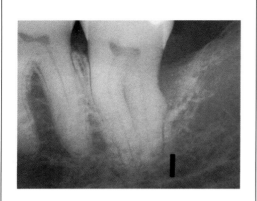

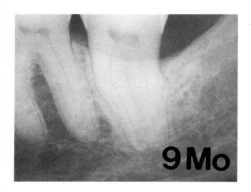

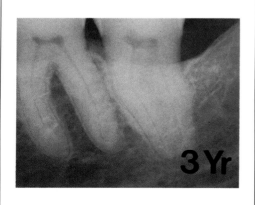

Fig 8-4h to j    Initial, 9-month, and 3-year post-treatment radiographs. Note improvement in bone levels.

Table 8-1    Clinical measurements of recession, probing depth, and clinical attachment level for three-walled intrabony defects

| Examination time | Probing depth (mm) | Attachment level (mm) |
|---|---|---|
| Initial | 9.43 | 9.01 |
| 9 mo | 2.78 | 4.48 |
| 3 y | 3.25 | 4.35 |

# Root conditioning with GTR procedures

The influence of the root surface in the regenerative process has resulted in several studies relating to root conditioning and GTR procedures. Gottlow et al (1984b) placed periodontitis-involved roots into contact with gingival connective tissue and bone. Half of the roots were treated with citric acid and the remaining roots served as controls. New attachment did not occur on either the citric acid–treated roots or the controls. Healing was mainly by root resorption and ankylosis.

Peterson and Aukhil (1986) created experimental fenestration wounds in an animal model. Half of the roots received root conditioning and a Millipore filter, while the control sites received only filters. New attachment formed on the control and test roots; however, acid-treated roots had greater resorption.

Garrett et al (1988) treated various types of osseous defects in 21 patients. The roots received citric acid conditioning prior to placement of either demineralized freeze-dried bone grafts or freeze-dried dura mater. The results from the three methods of treatment produced modest improvement in the clinical measurements.

Schallhorn and McClain (1988) cleaned the roots with citric acid before placing composite bone grafts and membranes over various osseous defects. No attempts were made to burnish the acid into the roots. Although no controls were used, the acid-treated roots together with bone grafting and membrane placement appeared to show the greatest improvement in clinical probing depth and attachment level.

Recently Handelsman and coworkers (1991) reported on a controlled study that compared citric acid–treated roots and membrane placement to nontreated roots and membrane placement. The defects were primarily deep combination two- and three-walled and three-walled intrabony lesions. The sites that received citric acid showed a mean decrease in probing depth of 4.9 mm and an average gain of clinical attachment of 3.5 mm. The sites that received only debridement and membrane placement had an average 5.4-mm decrease in probing depth and a mean 4.0-mm gain in clinical attachment. There was an average gain in bone level of 2.7 mm for defects treated with citric acid and an average bone increase of 3.8 mm for defects treated with debridement and membrane placement without acid treatment. The addition of root conditioning to the procedure did not appear to enhance changes in probing depth, attachment levels, or bone levels.

It appears that GTR procedures can be successfully used to improve clinical probing depth, attachment levels, and bone levels in deep multiwalled intrabony defects. Class II furcations with vertical components can likewise be successfully treated. New attachment procedures for class III furcation involvements require further research and refinement of surgical techniques.

# References

American Academy of Periodontology. Glossary of periodontic terms. *J Periodontol* 1986;57(suppl):19.

Aukhil I, Simpson DM, Schaberg TV. An experimental study of new attachment procedure in beagle dogs. *J Periodont Res* 1983;18:643–654.

Becker W, Becker BE, Berg L, Camsam C. Clinical and volumetric analysis of three-wall intrabony defects following open flap debridement. *J Periodontol* 1986a;57:277–285.

Becker W, Becker BE, Berg L. Repair of intrabony defects as a result of open debridement procedures. Report of 36 treated cases. *Int J Periodont Rest Dent* 1986b;6(2):9–21.

Becker W, Becker BE, Prichard J, et al. Root isolation for new attachment procedures. A surgical and suturing method: three case reports. *J Periodontol* 1987;58:819–826.

Becker W, Becker BE, Berg L, Prichard J, Caffesse R, Rosenberg E. New attachment after treatment with root isolation procedures: report for treated class III and class II furcations and vertical osseous defects. *Int J Periodont Rest Dent* 1988;8(3):9–23.

Blumenthal NM. The use of collagen membranes to guide regeneration of new connective tissue attachment in dogs. *J Periodontol* 1988;59:830.

Caffesse RG, Smith BA, Castelli WA, Nasjleti CE. New attachment achieved by guided tissue regeneration in beagle dogs. *J Periodontol* 1988;59:589–594.

Carranza FA. A technique for reattachment. *J Periodontol* 1954;25:272.

Caton J, Nyman S, Zander H. Histometric evaluation of periodontal surgery. II. Connective tissue attachment levels after four regenerative procedures. *J Clin Periodontol* 1980;7:224.

Ellegaard B, Karring T, Davis R, Löe H. New attachment after treatment of intrabony defects in monkeys. *J Periodontol* 1974;45:368.

Ellegaard B, Karring T, Löe H. New periodontal attachment procedure based on retardation of epithelial migration. *J Clin Periodontol* 1976;3:233.

Froum SJ, Coran J, Thaller B, et al. Periodontal healing following open debridement flap procedures. I. Clinical assessment of soft tissue and osseous repair. *J Periodontol* 1982;53:8.

Gara GG, Adams DE. Implant therapy in human intrabony pockets: a review of the literature. *J West Soc Periodontol Periodontal Abstr* 1981;29:32.

Gantes B, Martin M, Garrett S, Egelberg J. Treatment of periodontal furcation defects. (II) Bone regeneration in mandibular class II defects. *J Clin Periodontol* 1988;15:232.

Garrett S, Loos B, Chamberlain D, Egelberg J. Treatment of intraosseous periodontal defects with a combined adjunctive therapy of citric acid conditioning, bone grafting and placement of collagenous membranes. *J Clin Periodontol* 1988;15:383.

Goldman HM. A rationale for the treatment of the intrabony pocket: one method of treatment, subgingival curettage. *J Periodontol* 1949;20:83.

Goldman HM, Cohen DW. The intrabony pocket: classification and treatment. *J Periodontol* 1958;29:272.

Gottlow J, Nyman S, Karring T, Lindhe J. New attachment formation as the result of controlled tissue regeneration. *J Clin Periodontol* 1984a;11:494–503.

Gottlow J, Nyman S, Karring T. Healing following citric acid conditioning of roots implanted into bone and gingival connective tissue. *J Periodont Res* 1984b;19:214–220.

Gottlow J, Nyman S, Lindhe J, Karring T, Wennstrom J. New attachment formation in the human periodontium by guided tissue regeneration. Case reports. *J Clin Periodontol* 1986;13:604–616.

Handelsman M, Davapanah M, Celletti R. Guided tissue regeneration with and without citric acid treatment in vertical osseous defects. *Int J Periodont Rest Dent* 1991;11:303–315.

Hancock EB. Regeneration procedures. In: Nevins M, Becker W, Kornman K, eds. *Proceedings of the World Workshop in Clinical Periodontics.* Chicago: American Academy of Periodontology; 1989:VI-1–VI-20.

Iglhaut J, Aukhil I, Simpson DM, Johnson MS, Koch G. Progenitor cell kinetics during guided tissue regeneration on experimental periodontal wounds. *J Periodont Res* 1988;23:107.

Karring T, Isidor F, Nyman S, Lindhe J. Healing following implantation of periodontitis affected roots into bone tissue. *J Clin Periodontol* 1980;7:96–105.

Karring T, Nyman S, Lindhe J, Sirirat M. Potentials for root resorption during periodontal wound healing. *J Clin Periodontol* 1983;11:41–52.

Lorato DC. Intrabony defects in the dry human skull. *J Periodontol* 1970;41:496–498.

Magnusson I, Nyman S, Karring T, Egelberg J. Connective tissue attachment formation following exclusion of gingival connective tissue and epithelium during healing. *J Periodont Res* 1985;20:201–208.

Magnusson I, Batich C, Collins BR. New attachment formation following controlled tissue regeneration using biodegradeable membranes. *J Periodontol* 1987;59:1.

Melcher AH. On the repair potential of periodontal tissues. *J Periodontol* 1976;47:256.

Melcher AH, Cheong T, Cox J, Nemeth E, Shiga A. Synthesis of cementum-like tissue in vitro by cells cultured from bone: a light and electron microscopic study. *J Periodont Res* 1986;22:246.

Monson FD, Nichollson K. The distribution of bone defects in chronic periodontitis. *J Periodontol* 1974;45:88–92.

Nyman S, Karring T, Lindhe J, Planten S. Healing following implantation of periodontitis affected roots into gingival connective tissue. *J Clin Periodontol* 1980;7:394–401.

Nyman S, Gottlow J, Karring T, Lindhe J. The regeneration potential of the periodontal ligament. An experimental study in the monkey. *J Clin Periodontol* 1982a;9:257–265.

Nyman S, Lindhe J, Karring T. New attachment following surgical treatment of human periodontal disease. *J Clin Periodontol* 1982b;9:290–296.

Peterson EC, Aukhil I. Citric acid conditioning of roots affects guided tissue regeneration in experimental periodontal wounds. *J Periodont Res* 1986;21:543.

Pitaru S, Tal H, Soldinger M, Azar-Avidan O, Noff M. Collagen membranes prevent the apical migration of epithelium during periodontal wound healing. *J Peridont Res* 1987;22:331.

Pitaru S, Tal H, Soldinger M, Grosskopf A, Noff M. Partial regeneration of periodontal tissues using collagen barriers. Initial observations in the canine. *J Periodontol* 1988;59:380.

Polson AM, Heijl LC. Osseous repair in intrabony periodontal defects. *J Clin Periodontol* 1978;5:13.

Pontoriero R, Nyman S, Karring T, Rosenberg E, Sanavi F. Guided tissue regeneration in the treatment of furcation defects in man. *J Clin Periodontol* 1987;14:618.

Pontoriero R, Lindhe J, Nyman S, Karring T, Rosenberg E, Sanavi F. Guided tissue regeneration in degree II furcation-involved mandibular molars. A clinical study. *J Clin Periodontol* 1988;15:247.

Prichard JF. Regeneration of bone following periodontal therapy. *Oral Surgery* 1957a;10:247.

Prichard JF. The intrabony technique as a predictable procedure. *J Periodontol* 1957b;28:202.

Prichard JF. Treatment of intrabony pockets based on alveolar process after surgical intervention. *Dent Clin North Am* 1960;March:85.

Prichard JF. The diagnosis and management of vertical bony defects. *J Periodontol* 1983;54:29.

Renvert S, Badersten A, Nilveus R, Egelberg J. Healing after treatment of periodontal intra-osseous defects. I. Comparative study of clinical methods. *J Clin Periodontol* 1981;8:387–399.

Rosling B, Nyman S, Lindhe J. The effect of systematic plaque control on bone regeneration in intrabony pockets. *J Clin Periodontol* 1976;3:38.

Saari JT, Hurt WC, Biggs NL. Periodontal bony defects on the dry skull. *J Periodontol* 1968;39:278.

Schallhorn R, McClain PH. Combined osseous composite grafting, root conditioning, and guided tissue regeneration. *Int J Periodont Rest Dent* 1988;8(4):9.

Stahl SS, Froum SJ, Kushner L. Periodontal healing following open debridement flap procedures. II. Histologic observation. *J Periodontol* 1982;53:15.

Tal H, Lemmer J. Furcal defects in dry mandibles. *J Periodontol* 1982;53:364.

Tal H. Relationship between the depths of furcal defects and alveolar bone loss. *J Periodontol* 1982;53:631.

Tal H. The prevalence and distribution of intrabony defects in dry mandibles. *J Periodontol* 1984;55:149.

Winter G. Transcutaneous implant: reaction of the skin implant surface. *Biomed Mater Res Symp* 1974;5:99.

Chapter 9

# Resorbable Barriers and Periodontal Regeneration

Gary Greenstein / Jack G. Caton

Numerous reports have indicated that guided tissue regeneration (GTR) results in reduced probing depths and a gain of clinical attachment (Anderson 1991; Becker et al 1988; Caffesse et al 1990; Gottlow et al 1992; Greenstein and Caton 1990; Lekovic et al 1989; Paul et al 1992; Pontoriero et al 1988). These two objective clinical parameters were assessed to confirm that therapy arrests periodontal disease activity and induces repair of the periodontium. Since similar results have frequently been attained after conventional periodontal surgery, treatment outcomes that suggest GTR is better than conventional therapy need to be delineated.

In general, conventional treatment results in a 1-mm gain of clinical attachment (Greenstein1992), whereas GTR induces a 1.6- to 3.5-mm gain of clinical attachment (Becker et al 1988; Caffesse et al 1990; Gottlow et al 1992; Greenstein and Caton 1990; Lekovic et al 1989; Paul et al 1992; Pontoriero et al 1988). Histologic assessments have demonstrated that healing after conventional therapy is characterized by formation of a long junctional epithelium

(Caffesse et al 1988; Caton and Nyman 1980). Furthermore, surgical and nonsurgical techniques do not usually induce new connective tissue attachment. In contrast, GTR procedures facilitate partial regeneration of the periodontium to include new bone, cementum, and periodontal ligament (Aukhil et al 1986; Caffesse et al 1988; Minabe 1991).

Guided tissue regeneration is based on the biologic behavior of different tissues during healing. Barriers are placed subgingivally to exclude epithelium from migrating apically along the inner aspect of the flap. Barriers also prevent the undersurface of the flap, which is composed of connective tissue, from touching the root surface. Exclusion of cells from these two tissues facilitates progenitor cell migration from the periodontal ligament. However, questions have been raised whether improved periodontal status is induced by selective cell repopulation on a previously diseased root surface or to barrier protection and stabilization of the fibrin clot on the root (Magnusson et al 1990; Wikesjö et al 1991).

Overall, GTR procedures improve periodontal status, but histometric assessments reveal that incomplete regeneration frequently occurs (Aukhil et al 1986; Caffesse et al 1988; Magnusson et al 1990; Minabe 1991). For example, Aukhil et al (1986) noted three different zones of healing after barrier therapy: (1) junctional epithelium, (2) fibers parallel to the root surfaces, and (3) new connective tissue attachment (new bone, cementum, and periodontal ligament). Pitaru et al (1987) reported similar findings. They found regeneration of periodontal ligament, bone, and cementum in the apical half of defects, a long junctional epithelium in the coronal quarter, and a connective tissue adhesion between the two.

The guided tissue regeneration technique has the potential to regenerate varied amounts of lost periodontium in some defects. However, use of nonbiodegradable barriers dictates the need for secondary surgical procedures to remove the material. This is inconvenient for patients, is not cost effective, and is time-consuming for therapists. Barrier retrieval is a deterrent to routine use of GTR. To avoid secondary procedures, investigators have evaluated the efficacy of biodegradable materials to determine if they could provide results equivalent to nonbiodegradable barriers.

This paper reviews studies that assessed the utility of managing periodontal defects with resorbable barriers. The clinical and histologic findings are integrated into a discussion of whether biodegradable barriers provide the same benefits as nonresorbable barriers.

## Types of barriers

### Collagen

Collagen is natural protein and an integral part of mammalian tissues. There is a similarity between collagen in human skin and certain animal tissues. Since human body enzymes can degrade animal collagen, collagen is attractive as a barrier material. Furthermore, exogenous collagen is chemotactic for fibroblasts, enhances fibroblast attachment via its scaffoldlike fibrillar structure, and stimulates platelet degranulation, thereby accelerating fibrin and clot attachment (Blumenthal and Steinberg 1990; Lowenberg et al 1985; Pitaru et al 1987).

Initial studies to assess the efficacy of collagen were performed in dogs. Pitaru et al (1987, 1988, 1989) reported that rat collagen barriers could impede epithelial migration (Table 9-1). When test and control sites were compared, the amount of epithelial migration was reduced 50% by the barrier (test = 1.03 mm; control = 2.08 mm). There also was two times the amount of new connective tissue attachment (test = 1.6 mm; control = 0.8 mm) and more new bone and cementum at test sites. Barriers were resorbed after 30 days; however, their coronal edge (0.5 to 7 mm) was degraded within 10 days. The data were interpreted to indicate that the apical extent of epithelial migration was probably determined by the tenth postoperative day. These early studies by Pitaru et al established the potential for resorbable barriers to enhance periodontal regeneration.

It was suggested that limited results were possibly caused by barrier destruction induced by enzymes in plaque and healing wounds. To compensate for premature barrier degradation, Pitaru et al (1991) used bilayered collagen barriers. These provided an extra layer of collagen and the internal barrier was soaked with heparin sulfide and fibrin to attract progenitor cells. This resulted in a 95% root coverage with connective tissue cells, whereas monolayered and bilayered collagen without growth factors demonstrated 65% root coverage. These preliminary

Table 9-1    Resorbable barriers

| Study | Model (No. of subjects) | Defect | Barrier type | Length | Test | | Control |
|---|---|---|---|---|---|---|---|
| Blumenthal (1993) | Human | Furcation, class II | Collagen Gore-Tex | 12 mo | NA | 1.08 mm | — |
| | | | | | NA | 1.83 mm | — |
| Pitaru et al (1987) | Dog (3) | Dehiscence | Collagen | 10 d | EM | 0.34 mm | 0.82 mm |
| Pitaru et al (1988) | Dog (3) | Dehiscence | Collagen | 1 mo | EM | 1.03 mm | 2.08 mm |
| | | | | | NA | 1.6 mm | 0.8 mm |
| | | | | | NB | 1.92 mm | 0.2 mm |
| Pitaru et al (1990) | Dog (8) | Dehiscence | Collagen | 1 mo | NC | 2.2 mm | 0 mm |
| Blumenthal (1988) | Dog (4) | Two wall | Collagen | 3 mo | NA | 1.89 mm | 0.49 mm |
| Chung et al (1990) | Human (10) | 5 mm PD 40% bone loss | Collagen | 1 y | NA | 0.56 mm | −0.71 mm |
| | | | | | NB | 1.16 mm | 0 mm |
| Anderson (1991) | Human (18) | Furcation, class II | Collagen | 6 mo | NA | 0.33 mm | 0.79 mm |
| | | | | | NB | 1.63 mm | 0.30 mm |
| Quteish and Dolby (1992) | Human (19) | Various | Collagen | 6 mo | NA | 3.07 mm | 1.97 mm |
| Van Swol et al (1993) | Human (38) | Furcation, class II | Collagen | 3 mo | NA | 1.7 mm | 1.41 mm |
| | | | | | NB | 1.68 mm | .75 mm |
| Paul et al (1992) | Human (7) | Furcation, class II | Collagen | 6.9 mo | NA | 1.64 mm | 1.0 mm |
| | | | | | NB | 0.71 mm | 0.35 mm |
| Card et al (1989) | Dog (4) | Horizontal | Cargile | 3 mo | NC | 0.68 mm | −0.15 mm |
| | | | | | NB | 0.40 mm | −0.27 mm |
| Magnusson et al (1990) | Dog (8) | Circumferential palatal defects | PLA | 3 mo | NC | 2.1 mm | 2.1 mm |
| | | | | | NB | 1.1 mm | 1.1 mm |
| Gottlow et al (1992) | Humans (28) | Furcation, class II infrabony | PLA PLA | | NA | 3.2 mm | — |
| | | | | | NA | 4.9 mm | — |
| Warrer et al (1992) | Monkey (4) | Circumferential | PLA | 8 mo | NA | .7 mm | .5 mm |
| | | | | | NB | −.1 mm | −.1 mm |
| | | | Polyurethane | 8 mo | NA | .7 mm | .5 mm |
| | | | | | NB | .0 | −.1 mm |
| Polson et al (1993) | Human (9) | Furcation, class II | PLA | 6 mo | NA | 3.3 mm | — |
| Fleisher et al (1988) | Dog (1) | Dehiscence | Polyglactin | 77 d | NA | 80%–100% | 0%–25% |
| Quinones et al (1990) | Monkey (5) | Fenestration | Vicryl | 3 mo | NA | 100% | 100% |
| | | | | | NB | 100% | 100% |
| Quinones et al (1991) | Monkey (5) | Interproximal | Vicryl | 3 mo | NA | 83% | 8% |
| | | | | | NB | 72% | 11% |
| Caton et al (1990) | Human (10) | Furcation, class II | Vicryl | 6 mo | NA | 3.20 mm | 0.67 mm |
| Greenstein (1990) | Human (17) | Furcation, class II | Vicryl | 6 mo | NA | 2.64 mm | 0.7 mm |
| Kon et al (1992) | Dog (3) | Dehiscence | Gore-Tex Polyglactin | 85 d | | | |

| | GORE | POLY | Control |
|---|---|---|---|
| EM | 0.88 mm | 1.9 mm | 4.02 mm |
| NC | 2.82 mm | 1.1 mm | 0.24 mm |
| NA | 4.05 mm | 1.48 mm | 0.50 mm |

| Study | Model (No. of subjects) | Defect | Barrier type | Length | | MILL | PLA | Control |
|---|---|---|---|---|---|---|---|---|
| Magnusson et al (1988) | Dog (2) | Dehiscence | Millipore filter, PLA, control | 2 mo | NA | 25% | 46% | 12% |
| | | | | | | 1.4 mm | 2.5 mm | 0.7 mm |
| | | | | | NB | 1.7 mm | 2.1 mm | 0.8 mm |

*NA = new attachment (new attachment in humans refers to clinical attachment); NB = new bone; NC = new cementum; EM = epithelial migration; PLA = polylactic acid; MILL = Millipore filter; GORE = Gore-Tex Periodontal Material.

data suggested that barriers may enhance regeneration by providing a reservoir for chemotactic and attachment factors.

Blumenthal (1988) also used a dog model and reported that bovine collagen facilitated a modest gain of connective tissue attachment at test sites (1.89 mm) versus none at control sites. Barriers were eliminated at 8 weeks and there was little bone deposition. In contrast, when Blumenthal and Steinberg (1990) used a combination of bone grafting and collagen barrier, they reported that 93% of all defects achieved a 50% or greater fill of osseous defects. However, once again barriers as a monotherapy attained no bone fill.

Recently, several investigators have assessed the use of collagen barriers in a variety of defects in humans. Paul et al (1992) used resorbable type I bovine collagen in class II furcation defects. The material, Collistat (Vitaphore, Menlo Park, CA), is commercially available to facilitate hemostasis after surgical procedures. It is fully resorbable and has a half-life of 21 to 28 days when implanted in muscle. However, the investigators found that it frequently appeared to be absent 1 week after intraoral use. When barrier and conventional surgical therapy were compared, it was noted that barriers reduced probing depths better (1.5 versus 0.86 mm) and induced more horizontal bone formation (0.86 versus 0 mm). However, no differences were detected between test and control sites with regard to gain of clinical attachment or vertical defect fill. For most clinical parameters, these barriers provided no particular benefit.

Other studies conducted in humans provided more encouraging results when collagen barriers were used. Chung et al (1990) reported a gain of 0.56 mm of clinical attachment and 1.16 mm of new bone at test sites versus a loss of clinical attachment and no gain of bone at control sites. Similarly, Anderson et al (1991) demon-

strated partial regeneration of class II furcations with type I cross-linked collagen barriers (Table 9-1). Vertical bone fill was 1.63 mm at test sites versus 0.3 mm at control sites. However, clinical attachment gain was 0.33 mm (test) versus 0.79 mm for the control group. Conflicting data between bone fill and gain of clinical attachment indicate that additional studies are necessary to clarify the results.

Van Swol et al (1993) also reported that collagen barriers (Periogen, Collagen Corporation, Palo Alto, CA) improved periodontal status in the treatment of human class II furcations. He compared 28 patients with class II furcations who were treated with collagen membranes to 10 sham-operated controls. Membrane-treated defects demonstrated greater reduction of horizontal probing depths (2.28 mm versus 0.7 mm at control sites).

Relatively unsuccessful use of collagen barriers was reported by several investigators. Tanner et al (1988) found that Avitene (Alcon Laboratories, Fort Worth, TX), a microfibrillar collagen hemostat, was inefficient for retarding epithelial migration. Similarly, Pfeifer et al (1989) noted that non–cross-linked collagen barriers were not suitable for regenerative therapy because they resorbed within 3 weeks. However, cross-linked barriers were more successful because they did not resorb for 8 weeks. This latter paper was a descriptive report and no quantitative data were provided. When freeze-dried dura mater, a collagenous tissue, was used in human furcations, it did not improve periodontal status as well as grafts with coronally positioned flaps (Garrett et al 1988). The authors concluded that use of dura mater as a barrier provides no advantage over conventional therapy.

Certain materials such as rat collagen, Avitene, dura mater, and non–cross-linked collagen do not appear to provide a suitable environment for periodontal regeneration. The potential of other types of collagen to function as resorbable barriers has been demonstrated (Anderson 1991; Blumenthal 1988; Chung et al 1990; Van Swol 1991). However, there is no overwhelming evidence to suggest that collagen barriers predictably result in extensive regeneration of the periodontium when used in class II furcation defects or intrabony lesions. Furthermore, when Kobayashi et al (1991) compared Gore-Tex barriers (WL Gore & Assoc, Flagstaff, Ariz) to collagen membranes in a dog model, they noted that collagen membranes were only able to impede epithelial migration and failed to facilitate ingrowth of progenitor cells. Additional research is needed to determine if collagen barriers can provide more substantial and predictable results in periodontal defects.

## Oxidized cellulose

Galgut (1990) used oxidized cellulose mesh as a barrier. This commercially available resorbable hemostatic agent converts to a gelatinous mass upon incorporation with blood. The material was used in furcations and interdental infrabony defects in one patient. Galgut reported a reduction of probing depth and a gain of clinical attachment. This case report lacked any controls. Therefore, the improved periodontal status could not be attributed to GTR, because similar results were reported after conventional surgical procedures. In vivo and in vitro studies have indicated that this material resorbs without untoward effects, but additional research is needed to verify if oxidized cellulose has merit as a resorbable barrier.

## Cargile membranes

Only one study has used cargile membranes for GTR. Card et al (1989) used these membranes, which were prepared from the cecum of an ox, processed, and chromatized in a manner similar to suture material. The membranes were applied in dogs with naturally occurring periodontitis. Histologic assessment indicated that the barrier degraded in 4 to 8 weeks. Membranes deflected the epithelium, permitting significantly more new connective tissue (0.68 versus 0.15 mm) and bone (0.39 versus 0.27 mm) than did control sites. However, mean changes in probing depths and clinical attachment loss did not demonstrate any clinically significant differences. The investigators indicated that the material was difficult to manage and tended to fold over and stick to itself. Because the membranes were awkward to handle and results were limited, it was concluded that cargile membranes are not suitable for GTR.

## Hydrolyzable polyester

Caffesse and Nasjleti (1992) created defects in dogs and used a hydrolyzable polyester barrier. Barriers were well tolerated and produced minimal inflammatory response. Histometric data obtained after the animals were killed demonstrated greater new attachment (2.7 mm) and bone (1.7 mm) with increasing postoperative time. At 12 weeks the barriers began to disintegrate. The investigators concluded that this material has potential as a barrier in GTR. Additional controlled studies are needed to determine if hydrolyzable polyester will enhance regenerative procedures.

## Polylactic acid

Polylactic acid is a biodegradable ester polymer that was originally used in orthopedic surgery. Subsequently, Magnusson et al (1988) assessed the utility of polylactic acid barriers over buccal dehiscenes in dogs. They found a 2.5-mm gain of new cementum with inserting collagen fibers; this was equivalent to 40% of the initial defect. Control sites demonstrated regeneration in only 12% of induced defects. The authors

Table 9-2    Treatment of class II furcations in humans*

| Study | Probing depth reduction (mm) | Gain of clinical attachment (mm) | Recession (mm) | Barriers |
|---|---|---|---|---|
| Blumenthal (1993) | 2.67 | 1.08 | 1.59[†] | Gore-Tex |
| Paul et al (1992) | 1.5 | 1.64 | 0.14 | Collagen |
| Van Swol et al (1993) | 2.6 | 1.7 | 0.9 | Collagen |
| Caffesse et al (1990) | 2.80 | 1.8 | 1.0[†] | Gore-Tex |
| Blumenthal (1993) | 3.08 | 1.83 | 1.25[†] | Collagen |
| Becker et al (1988) | 3.30 | 2.3 | 1.30 | Gore-Tex |
| Greenstein & Caton (1990) | 3.86 | 2.64 | 1.05 | Vicryl mesh |
| Lekovic et al (1989) | 4.09 | 2.86 | 1.26 | Gore-Tex |
| Gottlow et al (1992) | 2.6 | 3.2 | —[‡] | Polylactic acid |
| Polson et al (1993) | 3.1 | 3.3 | .4 | Polylactic acid |
| Pontoriero et al (1988) | 4.0[§] | 3.5[§] | 0.5[†] | Gore-Tex |

*Arranged by increasing gain of clinical attachment.
[†]Calculated recession from data.
[‡]Data not reported.
[§]Average of buccal and lingual furcations.

noted that successful results were obtained after 2 months. Subsequently, Magnusson et al (1990) assessed polylactic acid in circumferential defects in dogs. There was 50% regeneration of connective tissue attachment in both test and control sites. These findings did not corroborate the previous study, which suggested that the barrier enhanced regenerative procedures.

Recently, a series of abstracts was published that provided additional support for the potential of polylactic acid as a resorbable barrier. Yamada et al (1991) evaluated polylactic acid membranes in a dog model. When test sites were compared to sham-operated control sites, it was noted that conventional surgery resulted in formation of a long junctional epithelium. At experimental sites, newly formed cementum covered 63% of the denuded roots.

Gottlow et al (1992) also attained favorable results with a bioabsorbable device (Guidor, John D. Butler Co, Chicago, Illinois) that was based on polylactic acid. Experimentally induced and treated defects in 12 monkeys demonstrated new attachment after 1 month, and bone formation was seen after 3 months. The barrier was totally

degraded by 6 months. The tissue compatibility of Guidor in humans was confirmed by Laurell et al (1992). The material was placed in 12 furcations and 20 infrabony defects. Recession was noted at 2 of 12 treated furcations and 11 of 20 infrabony defects. Recession averaged 2.2 mm (range of 1 to 5 mm). Probing depths were decreased from 5.6 to 3 mm in furcations and the mean gain of clinical attachment was 3.2 mm vertically and 3.1 mm horizontally. Complete closure of the furcation fornix was noted at 7 of 12 defects. Infrabony defects were reduced from 8.9 to 3.1 mm and there was a 4.9-mm gain of clinical attachment.

Assessment of the data in this last study indicated that furcations demonstrated a greater gain of clinical attachment than reduction of probing depth. This could only be accounted for by either coronal migration of the gingiva or measurement error. The finding that there was minimal or no recession contrasts with other investigations, which have routinely reported recession after barrier therapy (Table 9-2).

The preliminary data, which used crude barriers developed at chairside, was conflicting with regard to the efficacy of polylactic acid barriers (Magnusson et al 1988, 1990). However, recent abstracts have indicated that modifications of the polylactic acid barriers have increased their ability to enhance periodontal status (Gottlow et al 1992a, 1992b; Laurell et al 1992; Yamada et al 1991). Additional investigations are needed to assess the predictability of these barriers in a variety of different defects.

## Vicryl mesh (polyglactin 910)

Vicryl woven mesh is a synthetic material composed of glycolide and lactide in a 9:1 ratio, hence the name polyglactin 910. The material is processed and extruded as a fine filament and weaved into a mesh. The material has been used for sutures and in neurosurgery for many years.

Fleisher et al (1988) used vicryl barriers over created dehiscences on the buccal aspect of several teeth in one dog. Three sites that received a barrier demonstrated 80% to 100% connective tissue regeneration. Control sites only exhibited regeneration over 25% of the root surfaces.

In a monkey model, Quinones et al (1990) conducted a series of investigations using vicryl mesh to determine if it enhanced periodontal status at induced fenestration and interproximal defects. Histometric assessments revealed that after 1 month, fenestrated wounds treated with barriers demonstrated more new connective tissue attachment, bone, and developing ligament than did control sites. However, after 3 months both experimental and control sites manifested complete regeneration. The data were interpreted to indicate that vicryl mesh barriers promoted GTR. However, the finding of no differences at 3 months casts doubt on the clinical significance of the data. Interproximal defects in monkeys that received barriers exhibited thicker cementum, greater bone apposition, and a mature dense collagenous periodontal ligament after 3 months. In contrast, control sites manifested a long junctional epithelium with no further cementum or bone deposition (Quinones 1991).

A subsequent investigation in humans by Caton et al (1990) used vicryl barriers in class II furcation defects. The authors reported decreased vertical probing depths and a gain of clinical attachment when barrier-treated sites were compared to sham-operated control sites. Thirteen of 20 furcations were converted from class II (horizontal probing depth of 3 mm or more) to class I furcations (less than 3 mm).

As the number of sites included in the previous study were expanded, Greenstein and Caton (1990) reported 6-month data for 21 test and 17 control sites. They found that barrier-treated furcations, when compared to sham-operated controls, induced a greater probing depth reduction (3.86 versus 1.7 mm), a larger gain of clinical attachment (2.64 versus 0.7 mm) and an equivalent amount of recession (1.05 versus 1 mm) (Figs 9-1a to e). Horizontal probing depths were also reduced to a greater extent with barriers (3.7 to 2.4 mm) versus 3.1 to 3.1 mm at control sites. The mean data suggested that class II furcations were converted to class I furcations. However, in reality, 10 of 21 class II furcations persisted. Similarly, the mean values for the previously reported data did not adequately portray treatment responses. Approximately 70% to 80% of the treated sites had at least a 2-mm probing depth reduction and a 2-mm gain of clinical attachment. When these results were compared to findings reported for class II furcations after nonresorbable barriers were used, it appeared that the mean data attained with vicryl mesh was similar to the means reported in previous studies (see Table 9-2).

At sites that were reentered, there was little bone deposition, a finding that was consistent with other studies that assessed the effect of nonresorbable barriers in class II furcation defects. Furthermore, the fornix

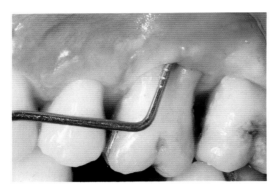

Fig 9-1a    Presurgical view of the maxillary left first molar, which had a class II buccal furcation and a vertical probing depth of 7 mm.

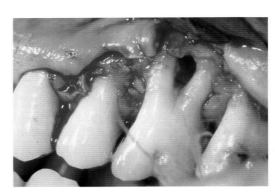

Fig 9-1b    The area after surgical debridement.

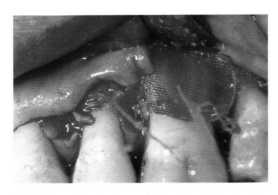

Fig 9-1c    A vicryl mesh barrier is ligated in place.

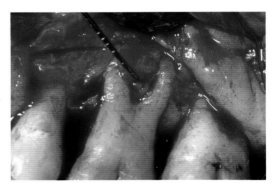

Fig 9-1d    At reentry 9 months postsurgery, the furcation is filled with dense connective tissue, no new bone is present, and the furcation fornix is probeable.

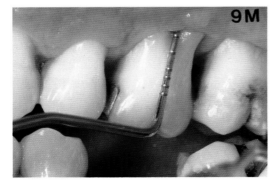

Fig 9-1e    Clinical appearance 9 months after reentry. The vertical probing depth is 2 mm and the furcation roof is probeable (2 mm).

of 16 of 21 furcations remained probeable and this was consistent with the results of other investigations (Becker et al 1987, 1988; Lekovic et al 1989).

Recently, Gager and Schultz (1991) reported that freeze-dried bone allograft used in conjunction with vicryl mesh enhanced osseous repair in interproximal defects. They demonstrated via a series of human case reports that combined therapy reduces probing depths and increases osseous fill, as assessed radiographically.

Results with vicryl mesh appear to be equivalent to results attained with nonresorbable barriers. However, the material has been tested in only a limited variety of defects, and defect elimination was often incomplete. Furthermore, it still needs to be determined if, when, and where allografts should be used in conjunction with vicryl mesh barriers (Figs 9-2a to h).

## Evidence and rationale for using resorbable barriers

There are several potential sources of progenitor cells during wound healing: epithelium, gingival connective tissue, alveolar bone, and periodontal ligament. To determine the contribution of each source, techniques were devised that excluded tissue components during wound maturation.

After conventional therapy, there appears to be a race between epithelial migration and coronal development of connective tissue. Epithelium migrates more quickly, resulting in formation of a long junctional epithelium without a gain of new connective tissue attachment. Therefore, to promote regeneration of the periodontium, it is necessary to retard epithelial invagination adjacent to previously diseased root surfaces. In this regard, the data in Table 9-1 indicate that sites where resorbable barriers were placed showed less epithelial migration. This was supported by direct histometric measurements of epithelial invagination (Kon et al 1991; Pitaru et al 1987, 1988) and indirect data that demonstrated biodegradable barriers resulted in more new cementum and connective tissue attachment than control sites (see Table 9-1). However, it was evident that most defects were incompletely resolved and were associated with variable amounts of epithelial migration. This is consistent with studies that assessed the efficacy of nonresorbable barriers (Aukhil et al 1986; Becker et al 1988; Caffesse et

al 1988, 1990; Lekovic et al 1989; Minabe 1991; Pontoriero et al 1988).

Investigators determined that connective tissue from the flap undersurface has the potential to induce root resorption (Karring et al 1980; Nyman et al 1980). Accordingly, barriers must ensure that gingival connective tissue does not contact the root surface until it is repopulated with progenitor cells or protected with a fibrin clot. Resorbable barriers appear to satisfactorily block out gingival connective tissue because root resorption has not been reported to any great extent (Blumenthal and Steinberg 1990; Fleisher et al 1988; Pitaru et al 1989; Quinones et al 1990, 1991).

Exclusion of epithelium and gingival connective tissue leaves two tissue compartments with potential to contribute progenitor cells—bone and the periodontal ligament. Determining the precise source of progenitor cells has been hampered because of lack of histologic and morphologic markers to identify cell type origin. Nevertheless, investigators have concluded that the periodontal ligament is the main source of progenitor cells because bone does not contribute to establishing connective tissue attachment (Gara and Adams 1981; Karring et al 1980). This was evident when roots were implanted within bone or when bone was implanted in defects contacting root surfaces.

Use of resorbable barriers usually results in formation of more new cementum, bone, and connective tissue attachment than does sham-operated control treatment (see Table 9-1). This attests to the fact that biodegradable barriers facilitate repopulation of root surfaces with progenitor cells from the periodontal ligament or are capable of protecting the fibrin clot.

At present, there appears to be a consensus that nonresorbable barriers do not have to remain in place more than 42 days (Caffesse 1992; Minabe 1991). Therefore, use of resorbable barriers that remain

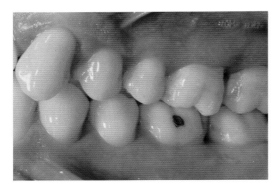

Fig 9-2a   Interproximal defects and 7-mm probing depth are present on the distal surfaces of both premolars.

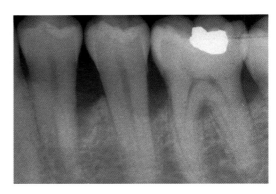

Fig 9-2b   The presurgical radiograph shows angular osseous defects on the distal surfaces of the premolars.

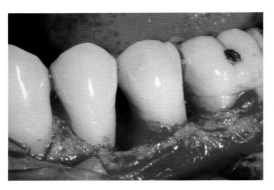

Fig 9-2c   Area after surgical debridement.

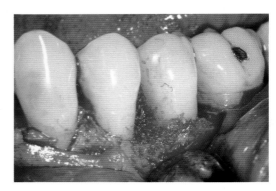

Fig 9-2d   Freeze-dried allograft placed in the defect of the first premolar. No bone was placed around the second premolar.

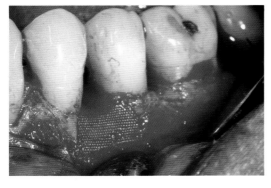

Fig 9-2e   Vicryl mesh barriers placed interproximally. The barriers were not ligated in place.

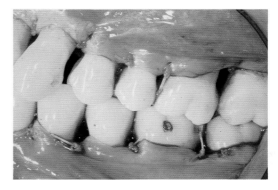

Fig 9-2f   The flaps are closed.

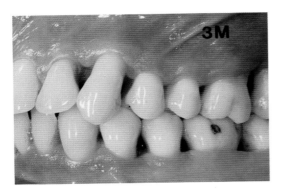

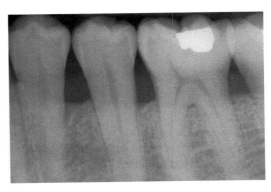

Fig 9-2g  Clinical view after 3 months. The vertical probing depth on the distal surfaces of the premolars is 2 to 3 mm.

Fig 9-2h  The radiograph taken after 12 months shows osseous deposition at the distal surfaces of both premolars.

Table 9-3  Time for resorption of barriers

| Study | Material | Model | Time (d) |
|---|---|---|---|
| Fleisher et al (1988) | Vicryl mesh | Dog | 30 |
| Quinones et al (1990) | Vicryl mesh | Monkey | 90 |
| Caton et al (1990) | Vicryl mesh | Human | 28–42 |
| Magnusson et al (1988) | Polylactic acid | Dog | 120 |
| Gottlow et al (1992a) | Polylactic acid | Human | <180 |
| Card et al (1989) | Cargile barriers | Dog | <60 |
| Caffesse & Nasjleti (1992) | Hydrolyzable polyester | Dog | 84 |
| Pitaru et al (1988) | Collagen | Dog | 28 |
| Blumenthal (1988) | Collagen | Dog | 64 |
| Van Swol et al (1993) | Collagen | Human | 70–84 |

intact for at least 6 weeks could fulfill this criterion and could preclude secondary surgical procedures to remove nonresorbable barriers. Many of the biodegradable barriers do not degrade for 6 weeks (Table 9-3). However, the time for resorption varies greatly among barriers and the models in which they are tested. In general, barriers are well tolerated by animals and humans, but sometimes the coronal edge of cargile and collagen barriers resorbs prematurely (Card et al 1989; Pitaru et al 1988). It appears that biodegradable barriers can function long enough to aid wound stabilization and/or promote selective repopulation of the root surface with progenitor cells. Additional investigations are needed to determine the ideal length of time that barriers should be present to maximize healing. Furthermore, it needs to be clarified whether barrier degradation interferes with wound healing.

## Healing of defects

Wide variability of results from tooth to tooth may be attributed to the type of defects being treated, duration of healing, type of barrier, and flap position (Caffesse et al 1988; Nyman et al 1987). Aukhil et al (1986) suggested that the extent of periodontal ligament regeneration may be limited because barrier placement creates two adjacent avascular walls (root and barrier). Thus the tissue must depend on an apical source for angiogenesis. This contention was supported by a previous report that revealed concomitant development of vascularity to be crucial for maximum migration of the periodontal ligament (Aukhil et al 1985). In this regard, incomplete healing is often noted after treatment of class II furcations in humans (Becker et al 1988; Caffesse et al 1990; Greenstein and Caton 1990; Lekovic et al 1989; Paul et al 1992), but some investigators reported a high percentage of furcation closure (Gottlow et al 1992a; Pontoriero et al 1988). Most studies indicated a gain of clinical attachment; however the roofs of furcations remain probeable. This is evident for both nonresorbable and resorbable barriers. Furthermore, most investigations noted that bone development is very limited or absent in treated furcations. Once again, this is true for biodegradable and nonbiodegradable barriers.

Several lines of evidence suggest that regeneration of bone and new connective tissue attachment progress independently. For example, bone fill occurs in angular defects opposite a long junctional epithelium after conventional therapy (Caton et al 1980; Listgarten and Rosenberg 1979). Similarly, in root implantation studies, the proximity of bone does not favor regeneration of new connective tissue attachment (Karring et al 1980; Nyman et al 1980). Conversely, it appears that the level of connective tissue attachment has no effect on bone repair. Lindhe et al (1984) demonstrated that if the periodontal ligament is left intact after buccal plate removal, a long supra-alveolar connective tissue attachment develops without appreciable bone apposition. Furthermore, Nyman et al (1980) reported the length of connective tissue attachment is not a determining factor for coronal regeneration of bone.

Others also demonstrated that new connective tissue attachment can form without concomitant bone deposition (Houston et al 1985; Karring et al 1985; Lindhe et al 1984). The finding that biodegradable and nonresorbable barriers induce a gain of clinical attachment with limited or no new bone is consistent with the concept that regeneration of bone and connective tissue attachment occur independently.

There are conflicting views in the literature with regard to the potential of different-sized defects to heal. Neiderman et al (1989) considered it a paradox that the greatest bone fill after barrier therapy was seen in large defects. It could be argued that these sites had the largest potential for fill, but the percentage of repair at these sites was greater than that for smaller lesion sites. In contrast, Pontoriero et al (1989) reported that larger defects had a smaller chance to attain furcation closure. They noted that wide-shallow defects had a better chance for healing than deep-narrow defects. This was attributed to the amount of remaining periodontal ligament that could provide progenitor cells. They concluded that defect size may be a factor and that the more periodontium, the greater the potential for new attachment to develop.

A variety of periodontal lesions were treated with resorbable barriers (see Table 9-1). However, no studies directly addressed the response of differently sized defects. At present, it is reasonable to conclude that several types of resorbable barriers (ie, vicryl mesh, collagen, polylactic acid) have the ability to enhance periodontal status in furcations and intrabony defects. However, their potential to induce regeneration in severe defects (ie, class III furcation) needs to be investigated.

## Wound stabilization

Current research has focused on two explanations regarding the biologic mecha-

Table 9-4    Comparative analysis: Resorbable versus nonresorbable barriers

| Study | Barrier type | | Comments |
|-------|--------------|--------------|----------|
|       | Resorbable | Nonresorbable | |
| Magnusson et al (1988) | Polylactic acid | Millipore filter | 46% regeneration—polylactic acid<br>25% regeneration—Millipore filter |
| Kon et al (1991) | Vicryl mesh | Gore-Tex | Gore-Tex was better (*see* Table 1) |
| Zappa & Caton (1992) | Vicryl mesh | Gore-Tex | Vicryl resulted in less horizontal furcation depth |
| Kobayashi et al (1991) | Collagen | Gore-Tex | Both retard epithelium; only Gore-Tex induced new connective tissue attachment |
| Galgut et al (1991) | Polylactic acid | Gore-Tex | Polylactic acid inhibited epithelium better than did Gore-Tex |
| Table 9-2* | Vicryl mesh<br>Polylactic acid | Gore-Tex | Equivalent results |

*See Table 9-2 in this chapter.

nism that facilitates regeneration of lost periodontium. Successful GTR is usually attributed to guided cells that repopulate a previously diseased root surface. However, another aspect of healing is stabilization of the root-clot interface.

Magnusson et al (1990) suggested that variations in healing related to differences in experimental defects cast doubt on the ability of GTR to resolve all defects. They hypothesized that healing is possibly caused by flap support or maintenance of space for clots. Barriers may supply support to the replaced flap, thus facilitating healing (Claffey et al 1989), and may protect the blood clot and its adherence to the root surface (Wikesjö et al 1991). The clot may be responsible for preventing apical migration of the junctional epithelium, allowing undisturbed wound maturation.

Polson and Proye (1983) examined the relationship between the coagulum and the root surface. They noted its fragile nature and concluded that coagulum stabilization is an important facet of wound repair. In this regard, resorbable barriers that are present during the early phases of wound repair can protect the fibrin clot from disruptive tensile forces. It takes several weeks before the root surface–gingival flap interface reaches sufficient maturity to withstand tissue manipulation (Wikesjö et al 1992). The few studies that assessed healing at different time points were interpreted to indicate that the critical phase of healing occurs within the first 2 months (Card et al 1989; Magnusson et al 1988, 1990; Pitaru et al 1989). Therefore, resorbable barriers that remain intact for 6 weeks appear to be able to fulfill the requirements of wound stabilization.

## Comparative analysis: resorbable and nonresorbable barriers

Table 9-4 lists studies that compared resorbable and nonresorbable barriers and includes comments regarding the investigators' conclusions. The data in Table 9-2 suggest that vicryl mesh and polylactic acid barriers attained results equivalent to those obtained by nonresorbable barriers. At present, it is not possible to determine if resorbable barriers are superior to nonresorbable barriers (or vice versa) for enhancing periodontal regeneration.

To date, no studies have directly compared the efficacy of different resorbable barriers. Comparison of biodegradable barriers in different investigations is difficult because of dissimilar defect morphologies and animal models. Nevertheless, it can be surmised that the resorbable barriers with the greatest potential to induce regeneration are vicryl mesh, polylactic acid, and collagen barriers.

Several features of resorbable barriers appear to be consistent with nonresorbable barriers. Results from human clinical trials indicate that barrier therapy usually resulted in more than twice as much gain of clinical attachment than did control treatment (see Table 9-1). Histometric data in animals confirmed that sites receiving resorbable barriers usually attained two to three times the amount of new connective tissue attachment observed at control sites. Furthermore, it appears that it is difficult to close the roofs of furcations.

## Conclusions

Overall, therapy with resorbable or nonresorbable barriers improves periodontal status but does not predictably result in complete regeneration of defects. However, barrier use is usually able to convert teeth with questionable prognoses into ones that are more easily maintainable. Additional investigations are needed to assess the benefits of using resorbable barriers in combination with graft materials, root surface conditioning agents, and growth factors. In the near future, clinicians may be able to predictably regenerate lost periodontium.

## References

Anderson HH. The effectiveness of a collagen membrane barrier in achieving new attachment in class II furcations. *J Periodontol* 1991;62:718.

Aukhil I, Iglhaut J, Suggs C, et al. An in vivo model to study migration of cells and orientation of connective tissue fibers in simulated periodontal spaces. *J Periodont Res* 1985;20:392–402.

Aukhil I, Petersson E, Suggs C. Guided tissue regeneration. An experimental procedure in beagle dogs. *J Periodontol* 1986;57:727–734.

Becker W, Becker BE, Prichard JF, et al. Root isolation for new attachment procedures. A surgical and suturing method: three case reports. *J Periodontol* 1987;58:819–826.

Becker W, Becker B, Berg L, et al. New attachment after treatment with root isolation procedures: report for treated class III and class II furcations and vertical osseous defects. *Int J Periodont Rest Dent* 1988;8(3):2–16.

Blumenthal NM. The use of collagen membranes to guide regeneration of new connective tissue attachment in dogs. *J Periodontol* 1988;59:830–836.

Blumenthal NM, Steinberg J. The use of collagen membrane barriers in conjunction with combined demineralized bone collagen gel implants in human infrabony defects. *J Periodontol* 1990;61:319–327.

Blumenthal NM. A clinical comparison of collagen membranes with e-PTFE membranes in the treatment of human mandibular buccal class II furcation defects. *J Periodontol* 1993;64:925–933.

Caffesse RG, Smith BA, Castelli WA, Nasjleti CE. New attachment achieved by guided tissue regeneration in beagle dogs. *J Periodontol* 1988;59:589–594.

Caffesse RG, Smith AB, Duff B, et al. Class II furcations treated by guided tissue regeneration in humans: case reports. *J Periodontol* 1990;61:510–514.

Caffesse RG. GTR: biologic rationale, surgical technique, and clinical results. *Compend Contin Educ Dent* 1992;8:166–178.

Caffesse RG, Nasjleti CE. Response to an absorbable membrane for guided tissue regeneration in dogs. *J Dent Res* 1992;71:297(abstr no. 1534).

Card SJ, Caffesse RG, Smith B, Nasjleti C. New attachment following the use of a resorbable membrane in treating periodontitis in beagle dogs. *Int J Periodont Rest Dent* 1989;9:59–69.

Caton J, Nyman S. Histometric evaluation of periodontal surgery. I. The modified Widman flap procedure. *J Clin Periodontol* 1980;7:212–223.

Caton J, Nyman S, Zander H. Histometric evaluation of periodontal surgery. Part II: Connective tissue attachment levels after four regenerative procedures. *J Clin Periodontol* 1980;7:224–231.

Caton J, Frantz B, Greenstein G, et al. Synthetic biodegradable barrier for regeneration in human periodontal defects. *J Periodont Res* 1990;69:275(abstr no. 1335).

Claffey N, Mostinger S, Ambruster J, Egelberg J. Placement of a porous membrane underneath the mucoperiosteal flap and its effect on periodontal wound healing in dogs. *J Clin Periodontol* 1989;16:12–16.

Chung KM, Salkin LM, Stein MD, Freedman AL. Clinical evaluation of a biodegradable collagen membrane in guided tissue regeneration. *J Periodontol* 1990;61:732–736.

Fleisher N, Waal HD, Bloom A. Regeneration of lost attachment apparatus in the dog using vicryl absorbable mesh (Polyglactin 910). *Int J Periodont Rest Dent* 1988;8(2):45–54.

Gager AH, Schultz AJ. Treatment of periodontal defects with an absorbable membrane (Polylactin 910) with and without osseous grafting. *J Periodontol* 1991;62:276–283.

Galgut PN. Oxidized cellulose mesh used as a biodegradable barrier membrane in the technique of guided tissue regeneration. A case report. *J Periodontol* 1990;61:766–768.

Galgut P, Pitrola R, Waite I, et al. Histologic evaluation of biodegradable and non-degradable membrane placed transcutaneously in rats. *J Clin Periodontol* 1991;18:581–586.

Gara GG, Adams DF. Implant therapy in human intrabony defects: a review of the literature. *J West Soc Periodontol-Periodont Abstr.* 1981;29:32–47.

Garrett S, Loos B, Chamberlain D, Egelberg J. Treatment of intraosseous periodontal defects with a combined adjunctive therapy of citric acid conditioning, bone grafting, and placement of collagenous membranes. *J Clin Periodontol* 1988;15:383–389.

Gottlow J, Nyman S, Laurell L, et al. Clinical result of GTR-therapy using a bioabsorbable device (Guidor). *J Dent Res* 1992a;71:298(abstr no. 1536).

Gottlow J, Lundgren D, Nyman S, et al. New attachment formation in the monkey using Guidor, a bioabsorbable GTR-device. *J Dent Res* 1992b;71:297(abstr no. 1535).

Greenstein G, Caton J. Treatment of class II furcation involvements with woven vicryl mesh. Presented at the Annual Meeting of the American Academy of Periodontology, Dallas, Texas, Oct 1990.

Greenstein G. Periodontal response to mechanical non-surgical therapy. A review. *J Periodontol* 1992;63:118–130.

Houston F, Sarhed G, Nyman S, Lindhe J. Healing after tooth reimplantation in monkeys. *J Clin Periodontol* 1985;12:728–735.

Karring T, Nyman S, Lindhe J. Healing following implantation of periodontitis affected roots into bone tissue. *J Clin Periodontol* 1980;7:96–105.

Karring T, Isidor E, Nyman S, Lindhe J. New attachment formation on teeth with a reduced but healthy periodontal ligament. *J Clin Periodontol* 1985;12:51–60.

Kobayashi H, Goultschin J, Caffesse RG, et al. Histologic response to collagen barriers in guided tissue regeneration. *J Dent Res* 1991;70:507(abstr no. 1926).

Kon S, Ruben M, Bloom A, et al. Regeneration of periodontal ligaments using resorbable and nonresorbable membranes: clinical, histological and histometric study in dogs. *Int J Periodont Rest Dent* 1991;11:59–71.

Laurell L, Gottlow J, Nyman S, et al. Gingival response to Guidor, a biodegradable device in GTR-therapy. *J Dent Res* 1992;71:298(abstr no. 1536).

Lekovic V, Kenney EB, Kovacevic K, Carranza FA. Evaluation of guided tissue regeneration in class II furcation defects. A clinical reentry study. *J Periodontol* 1989;60:694–698.

Lindhe J, Nyman S, Karring T. Connective tissue reattachment as related to the presence or absence of alveolar bone. *J Clin Periodontol* 1984;11:33–40.

Listgarten MA, Rosenberg MM. Histological study of repair following new attachment procedures in human periodontal lesions. *J Periodontol* 1979;50:333–344.

Lowenberg BF, Aubin JE, Deporter DA, et al. Attachment, migration and orientation of human gingival fibroblasts to collagen coated, surface demineralized, and untreated root slices. *J Dent Res* 1985;64:(abstr no. 1106).

Magnusson I, Batich C, Collins BR. New attachment formation following controlled tissue regeneration using biodegradable membranes. *J Periodontol* 1988;59:1–7.

Magnusson I, Stenberg WV, Batich C, Egelberg J. Connective tissue repair in circumferential periodontal defects in dogs following use of a biodegradable membrane. *J Clin Periodontol* 1990;17:243–248.

Minabe M. Critical review of the biologic rationale for guided tissue regeneration. *J Periodontol* 1991;62:171–179.

Neiderman R, Savit ED, Heeley JD, Duckworth JE. Regeneration of furca bone using Gore-Tex periodontal material. *Int J Periodont Rest Dent* 1989;9:469–480.

Nyman S, Karring T, Lindhe J. Healing following implantation of periodontitis roots into gingival connective tissue. *J Clin Periodontol* 1980;7:394–401.

Nyman S, Gottlow J, Lindhe J, et al. New attachment formation by guided tissue regeneration. *J Periodont Res* 1987;22:252–254.

Paul B, Mellonig JT, Towle HJ, Gray LJ. Use of a collagen barrier to enhance healing in human periodontal furcation defects. *Int J Periodont Rest Dent* 1992;12:123–131.

Pfeifer J, Van Swol R, Ellinger R. Epithelial exclusion and tissue regeneration using a collagen membrane barrier in chronic periodontal defects. A histologic study. *Int J Periodont Rest Dent* 1989;9:263–274.

Pitaru S, Tal H, Soldinger M, Azar-Avidam O, Noff M. Collagen membrane prevents the apical migration of epithelium during periodontal wound healing. *J Periodont Res* 1987;22:331–333.

Pitaru S, Tal H, Soldinger M, Grosskopf A, Noff M. Partial regeneration of periodontal tissues using collagen barriers. Initial observations in the canine. *J Periodontol* 1988;59:380–386.

Pitaru S, Tal H, Soldinger M, Noff M. Collagen membrane prevent apical migration of epithelium and support new connective tissue during periodontal wound healing in dogs. *J Periodont Res* 1989;24:247–253.

Pitaru S, Noff M, Grosskopf A, et al. Heparin sulfate and fibronectin improve the capacity of collagen barriers to prevent apical migration of the junctional epithelium. *J Periodontol* 1991;628:598–601.

Polson AM, Proye MP. Fibrin linkage. A precursor for new attachment. *J Periodontol* 1983;54:141–147.

Polson AM, Southard GL, Dunn RL, Polson AP, Billin JR. Initial study of GTR in class II furcation defects after using a biodegradable barrier [research forum]. Annual American Academy of Periodontology meeting, October 1993.

Pontoriero R, Lindhe J, Nyman S, et al. Guided tissue regeneration in degree II furcation involved mandibular molars. A clinical study. *J Clin Periodontol* 1988;15:247–254.

Pontoriero R, Lindhe J, Nyman S, et al. Guided tissue regeneration in the treatment of furcation defects in mandibular molars. A clinical study of degree III involvements. *J Clin Periodontol* 1989;16:170–174.

Quiñones CR, Caton JG, Polson AM, et al. Evaluation of synthetic biodegradable barriers to facilitate guided tissue regeneration. *J Periodont Res* 1990;69:275(abstr no. 1336).

Quiñones CR, Caton JG, Polson AM, et al. Evaluation of synthetic biodegradable barriers to facilitate guided tissue regeneration in interproximal sites. *J Periodontol* 1991;62:86(abstr).

Quteish D, Dolby AE. The use of irradiated-cross linked human collagen membrane in guided tissue regeneration. *J Clin Periodontol* 1992;19:476–484.

Tanner M, Solt CW, Vudhakanok S. An evaluation of new attachment formation using a microfibrillar collagen barrier. *J Periodontol* 1988;59:524–530.

Van Swol R, Ellinger R, Pfeiffer J, Barton NE, Blumenthal N. Collagen membrane barrier therapy to guide regeneration in class II furcations in humans. *J Periodontol* 1993;64:622–629.

Warrer K, Karring T, Nyman S, Gogolewski S. Guided tissue regeneration using biodegradable membranes of polylactic acid or polyurethane. *J Clin Periodontol* 1992;19:633–640.

Wikesjö UME, Claffey N, Egelberg J. Periodontal repair in dogs: effect of heparin treatment on the root surface. *J Clin Periodontol* 1991;18:60–64.

Wikesjö UME, Nilveus RE, Selvig KA. Significance of early healing events in periodontal repair: a review. *J Periodontol* 1992;63:158–165.

Yamada S, Takahashi Y, Matsumoto Y, et al. The use of polylactic acid membrane in guided tissue regeneration in dogs. *J Dent Res* 1991;70:507(abstr no. 1928).

Zappa U, Caton J. Non-resorbable and biodegradable barriers for regeneration in human periodontal defects. *J Dent Res* 1992;72:623(abstr no. 861).

# Chapter 10

# Cellular and Molecular Biology of Periodontal Wound Healing

Victor P. Terranova / Ray M. Price / Fusanori Nishimura / Jiuming Ye

Adult periodontitis may have its onset in adolescence and continue for the life of the individual. It is usually not clinically significant until the patient reaches middle age. Prevalence and severity increase with age; progress of the disease is generally slow and continuous when evaluated by pooled data, and there appears to be no sex predilection (Loesche 1982). Previous studies have indicated that the presence and severity of adult periodontitis is directly related to the presence of long-standing plaque and calculus (Loesche 1982; Tanner et al 1979). The initiation of the disease and the subsequent conversion of an established lesion to an advanced lesion (periodontitis), characterized by destruction of the connective tissue attachment to the root surface, has been studied, but the biologic mechanisms involved are not understood (Loesche 1982; Tanner et al 1979). There are few published studies that address the biologic, biochemical, and molecular biologic events necessary to repair the destruction once the destructive disease has been initiated. The Laboratory of Tumor Biology and Connective Tissue Research has made substantial progress in defining some of these events with special emphasis on the cellular and molecular biology.

## Biologic basis of repair

Recent clinical investigations with focus on regeneration of the periodontium have attempted to define factors involved in the formation of a new connective tissue attachment to periodontally diseased or denuded root surfaces (Selvig 1983; Terranova et al 1986, 1987). One essential biologic event involved in tissue regeneration is specific cell-directed migration (chemotaxis). Chemotaxis is an essential feature of many biologic processes in health and disease. Examples are ectodermal cell migration in development, movement of endothelial cells in the process of neovascularization, movement of fibroblasts in wound healing, neurite outgrowth, movement of polymorphonuclear leukocytes to areas of infection, movement of smooth muscle cells in atherosclerosis, and movement of tumor cells to form metastases (Akers et al 1981; Azizkhan et al

1980; Gaus-Muller et al 1980; Grotendorst et al 1981; McCarthy and Furcht 1984; McCarthy et al 1983; Schiffmann and Gallin 1979; Seppa et al 1982; Terranova et al 1985).

Both fibronectin and laminin and certain proteoglycans have been implicated in the directed movement of different cell types. Other extracellular matrix proteins or fragments of larger molecules have also been shown to possess chemotactic properties (Terranova and Lyall 1986). In addition, growth factors (polypeptide mitogens) have recently been reported to be chemotactic for various cell types. The extended form of b-FGF (basic fibroblast growth factor) has been shown to be a potent chemoattractant for human endothelial cells (Terranova et al 1985). Other growth factors that have been shown to possess chemoattractant activity include PDGF (platelet-derived growth factor), NGF (nerve growth factor), EGF (epidermal growth factor), and TGF-$\alpha$ and TGF-$\beta$ (transforming growth factors alpha and beta) (Terranova and Lyall 1986; Terranova and Wikesjö 1988).

The repair of injury begins as soon as tissue damage occurs. The release of polypeptide growth factors from injured cells and inflammatory cells is a critical part of the repair process. Many of the polypeptide growth factors have been shown to be involved in tissue repair (Sporn and Roberts 1986). For example, PDGF, TGF-$\alpha$, and TGF-$\beta$ are three polypeptides that have been shown to play an important role. PDGF is initially released from the alpha-granules of platelets and is a potent mitogen for fibroblasts in the presence of either TFG-$\alpha$ or EGF (Deuel et al 1985; Ross et al 1986). Furthermore, PDGF stimulates the production of both types I and IV collagenase (recently shown to be chemotactic for endothelial cells) by fibroblasts and thus contributes to the remodeling of matrix components, an essential feature of tissue repair. Peptides resembling TFG-$\alpha$ have

been found in platelets, activated macrophages, and in the ascites fluid of cirrhotic patients. TGF-$\alpha$, with its high degree of homology to EGF and to the B2 chain of laminin, has been shown to be very important for the growth potential and integrity of most epidermal cells (Assoian and Sporn 1986). TGF-$\beta$ appears to have a particularly important role in the repair process. This peptide is found in relatively high concentrations in platelets, in activated T lymphocytes, as well as in macrophages. TGF-$\beta$ stimulates the formation of collagen in humans or rodent fibroblasts and when injected subcutaneously in newborn mice causes rapid fibrotic and angiogenic response at the site of injection. Another recently discovered source of TGF-$\beta$ is bone. Transforming growth factor beta is present in bone in amounts almost 100-fold greater than those found in soft tissues and has some degree of homology with the BMP-2A (bone morphogenic protein-2A), BMP-2B, and BMP-3. In vitro studies indicate that TGF-$\beta$ can control the effects of several other polypeptide growth factors including PDGF, TGF-$\alpha$, EGF, a-FGF, b-FGF, and IL-2 (interleukin 2) (Assoian et al 1984; Bowen-Pope and Seifert 1985; Kehrl et al 1986; Mehlman and Maciag 1985; Seyedin et al 1986). To fully understand the mechanism of action of these peptide growth factors it must be realized that they act in sets or combinations in which each peptide modulates the effects of the next peptide.

Although there may be an autocrine action of these peptides in injured cells, it would appear that their paracrine action, driven by their production and release by various inflammatory cells, accounts for the key role of these peptides in the repair process (Bowen-Pope and Seifert 1985; Kehrl et al 1986; Mehlman and Maciag 1985). However, autocrine function may play an important role. This role has been demonstrated in traumatized cultures of arterial smooth muscle cells that synthesize and release peptides that resemble PDGF. The function of some of these known peptides in relationship to cells of the periodontium is presently under investigation (Terranova and Wikesjö 1988b). In addition, other factors isolated from cementum may have the potential to be mitogenic or chemotactic for cells of osseous or ligament origin.

Among the least understood aspects of generalized tissue repair are the combinations and temporal sequence of growth factors that initiate and control cell motility and proliferation. Possibly a unique autocrine factor is responsible for initiation of this event. Recently an autocrine motility factor (AMF) was identified for melanoma cells. This factor was found to be unique, based on amino acid analysis, and to have a molecular weight of 55,000 (Liotta et al 1986). Its action may be associated with membrane changes in phospholipid methylation. Similar membrane changes have been implicated in the motility of leukocytes. In other systems, marked increases in phospholipid methylation have been observed in hormonal effects on hepatocytes, adipocytes, and bladder epithelial cells.

By using a newly developed assay system, this laboratory is able to test the potential activity of various biologic response modifiers using dentin as a substrate. The assay system is divided into two parts. Assay I allows the measurement of the chemotactic activity of the test substance bound to dentin. Here the cells must actively move through a filter (eg, Nucleopore [Pledsanton,

CA], 100-$\mu$m thick, 8-$\mu$m pore diameter) in response to biologic response modifiers bound to dentin. In assay II, the ability of the dentin-bound factors to stimulate directed movement and proliferation of periodontal tissue cells on dentin surfaces are measured. Using these assays, we have demonstrated that human periodontal ligament cells migrate to fibronectin, PDGF, a-FGF, b-FGF, and TGF-$\beta$ (Table 10-1; Figs 10-1 and 10-2). In addition, fibronectin, PDGF, a-FGF, b-FGF, and TGF-$\beta$ induce a proliferative response in periodontal ligament cells grown on surface-demineralized dentin or in tissue culture (Table 10-2; Figs 10-3 to 10-5). Human gingival epithelial cells were shown to migrate to laminin, laminin fragments, and EGF (Table 10-3). Laminin was also shown to stimulate gingival epithelial cell proliferation on native dentin surfaces (Terranova et al 1986, 1987). These in vitro findings suggest that biologic conditioning of the root surface (dentin) may enhance mesenchymal cell attachment, migration, and proliferation. These events may subsequently lead to improved healing after periodontal reconstructive surgery.

The above-mentioned findings are not surprising because most, if not all, mesenchymal cells have receptors for the growth factors that have been examined. What was surprising was the lack of migration of periodontal ligament cells to TFG-$\alpha$ and EGF because cells of mesenchymal origin have been shown to have a limited number of receptors of high affinity for TGF-$\alpha$ (EGF) type molecules.

Table 10-1   Directed migration* of human periodontal ligament cells and human gingival fibroblasts

| Cell type | Biologic agents† | | | | | | |
|---|---|---|---|---|---|---|---|
| | FN | LM | a-FGF | b-FGF | NGF | PDGF | TBF-β |
| Human periodontal ligament cells | ++ | — | +++ | ++++ | 0 | ++ | ++++ |
| Human gingival fibroblasts | ++ | +/− | ++ | ++ | 0 | ++++ | +++ |

| Cell type | Combination of biologic agents | | |
|---|---|---|---|
| | PDGF + FGF | TGF-β + FN | FGF + TGF-β |
| Human periodontal ligament cell | ++++ | ++++ | ++++ |
| Human gingival fibroblasts | +++ | ++ | + |

*Chemotaxis assayed by counting the number of cells per high-power (×200) field.
†FN = fibronectin; LM = laminin; a-FGF, b-FGF = acidic or basic fibroblast growth factor; NGF = nerve growth factor; PDGF = platelet-derived growth factor; TGF-β = transforming growth factor.
0 No effect; — inhibitory; + Minimal effect; ++ Moderate stimulatory effect; +++ High stimulatory effect; ++++ Maximal stimulatory effect; +/− Subpopulations identified with both FN and LM receptors.

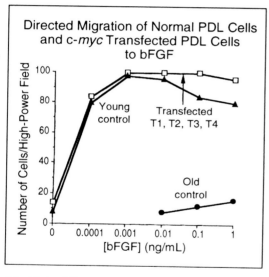

Fig 10-1   Migratory response of young and old periodontal ligament (PDL) cells to an increasing dose of bFGF. The four transfectants were also assayed for motility to bFGF.

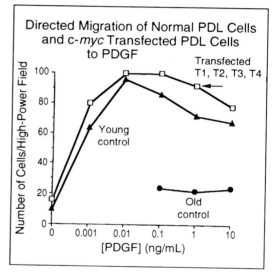

Fig 10-2   Migratory response of young and old periodontal ligament (PDL) cells to a dose-dependent increasing concentration of PDGF. The four transfectants were also assayed for motility to PDGF.

Table 10-2   Directed migration* of human gingival epithelial cells to various biologic agents

| Cell type | Biologic agents† | | | | | |
|---|---|---|---|---|---|---|
| | LM | EGF | TGF-α | b-FGF | NGF | TGF-β |
| Human gingival epithelial cells | ++++ | ++++ | ++++ | 0 | 0 | ++ |
| Human skin epithelial cells | ++++ | ++++ | ++++ | 0 | 0 | ++ |
| Human gingival fibroblasts | — | 0 | 0 | +++ | 0 | +++ |

*Chemotaxis assayed by counting the number of cells per high power field (×200).
†LM = laminin; EGF = epidermal growth factor; TGF-α = transforming growth factor alpha; b-FGF = basic fibroblast growth factor; NGF = nerve growth factor; TGF-β = transforming growth factor beta.
0 No effect; — inhibitory; + Minimal effect; ++ Moderate stimulatory effect; +++ High stimulatory effect; ++++ Maximal stimulatory effect.

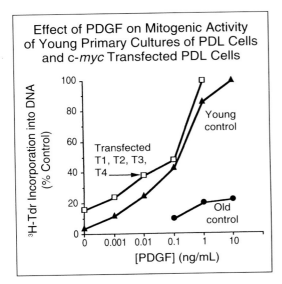

Fig 10-3   Dose response of ³H-Tdr incorporation of young and old periodontal ligament (PDL) cells in GFPS media with additions of PDGF (AB heterodimer, AA and BB homodimers); 100% incorporation of ³H-Tdr is equivalent to growth in 1% FBS. Additionally, four sets of c-*myc* transfected PDL cell lines (PDL-L1-T1[T2,T3,T4]) were compared.

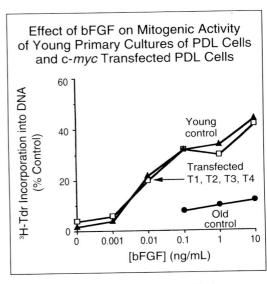

Fig 10-4   Dose response of ³H-Tdr incorporation for young and old periodontal ligament (PDL) cells in GFPS media with additions of bFGF; 100% incorporation is equivalent to growth in 1% FBS. Dose response of PDL-L1-T1(T2,T3,T4) is also shown.

In all of these studies, the basic premise has been to examine factors that could confer a selective advantage on periodontal ligament cells for stimulated adhesion, migration, and proliferation. What our studies have shown was that no one factor, alone or in combination with other factors, has the ability to uniquely stimulate periodontal ligament cells (see Table 10-1). Although the dose response profiles of the factors are different for different cell populations, the generalized results can be summarized as an all-or-none response. If we can assume that stimulation of only periodontal ligament cells is important in the initiating events in periodontal regeneration, then a periodontal ligament cell–specific (ligament-specific) factor is required. We make this suggestion based on the numbers of available cells that are anatomically positioned in the appropriate

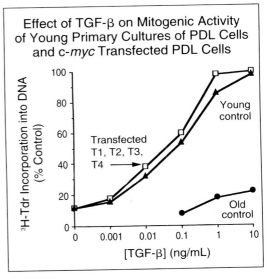

Fig 10-5   Dose response of ³H-Tdr incorporation into DNA for TGF-β stimulation of young, old, and c-*myc* transfected peridontal ligament (PDL) cells.

Table 10-3    Response of human periodontal ligament cells, human gingival fibroblast cells, and human gingival epithelial cells to different biologic agents that induce proliferation (% incorporation of $^3$H-TdR into DNA)*

| Cell type | Biologic agent[†] | | | | | |
|---|---|---|---|---|---|---|
| | FN | LM | PDGF[‡] | b-FGF | NGF | EGF |
| Human periodontal ligament cells | 30 | Cytotoxic | 100 | 60 | 10 | 15 |
| Human gingival fibroblasts | 46 | Cytotoxic | 100 | 65 | 5 | 10 |
| Human gingival epithelial cells | 0 | 100 | 100* | 15 | 25 | 100 |

*Percent incorporation of $^3$H-TdR into DNA based on incorporation of $^3$H-TdR into DNA using 1% fetal bovine serum as control and establishing this level as 100%. All experiments were performed in growth factor–poor serum. Baseline incorporation percentages are defined by $^3$H-TdR incorporation into DNA in cells previously washed with PBS for 48 hours after a double thymidine block to establish a synchronized population.
[†]FN = fibronectin; LM = laminin; PDGF = platelet derived growth factor; b-FGF = basic fibroblast growth factor; NGF = nerve growth factor; EGF = epidermal growth factor.
[‡]PDGF used in conjunction with either LM or EGF at various concentrations.

location for regeneration to occur. Connective tissue flaps contain numbers of mesenchymal cells several orders of magnitude greater than does the coronal exposure of the periodontal ligament. Additionally, the large number of activated epithelial cells exceeds periodontal ligament cell availability.

Is there in fact a periodontal ligament-specific factor? Our recent data indicate that there is a specific factor synthesized and secreted by periodontal ligament cells that is a chemotactic and mitogenic autocrine factor. These results were generated by examining conditioned media of periodontal ligament cells and of gingival fibroblasts and epithelial cells. When conditioned media from cultures of human periodontal ligament cells were examined for chemoattractant and mitogenic activity, we observed a dose-dependent relationship for periodontal ligament cells. Additional data suggested that a specific polypeptide found within the periodontal ligament cell–conditioned media is responsible for the biologic activity. Heating the media to 100°C for 30 minutes decreased the chemoattractant activity, as did a 60-minute incubation with trypsin. These two experiments indicated that the responsible factor has a polypeptide structure. Incu-

bation with other enzymes also eliminated the biologic activity. Gingival fibroblasts and epithelial cells did not respond to various concentrations of the periodontal ligament cell–conditioned media. These studies suggested a uniqueness of the factor that induces only periodontal ligament cell function. Antibodies against fibronectin and laminin as well as the FGF family or EGF and several cytokines did not inhibit the chemotactic or mitogenic properties of the conditioned media for periodontal ligament cells. Transforming growth factor beta enhances the activity of the periodontal ligament cell–conditioned media but antibodies directed against TGF-β did not inhibit the periodontal ligament factor–mediated chemotactic response observed using periodontal ligament cells. Reverse-phase high-pressure liquid chromatography (HPLC) has enabled us to isolate a 12,500-dalton peptide with high chemotactic and mitogenic activity (Table 10-4). Additional data from open-column chromatography and HPLC support the peptide nature of this material. Amino acid composition analysis and amino acid sequence data indicate a unique peptide. We have termed this factor PDL-CTX. In cell biology experiments, a subpopulation of periodontal ligament cells has been isolated. This

Table 10-4    Comparison of young and old periodontal ligament cells to various biologic agents

Chemotactic response (no. of cells per high power field)*

| Cell type | Biologic agent[†] | | | |
| --- | --- | --- | --- | --- |
| | FN | b-FGF | PDGF | PDL-CTX |
| Young periodontal ligament[‡] | ++ | ++++ | ++ | ++++ |
| Old periodontal ligament[§] | 0 | + | 0 | +++ |

Proliferative response (% VH=Tdr incorporation into DNA)[¶]

| Cell type | Biologic agent[†] | | | |
| --- | --- | --- | --- | --- |
| | FN | b-FGF | PDGF | PDL-CTX |
| Young periodontal ligament[‡] | 30 | 60 | 100 | 100(+) |
| Old periodontal ligament[§] | 5 | 5 | 10 | 80(+) |

*See Table 10-1 for description.
[†]FN = fibronectin; b-FGF = basic fibroblast growth factor; PDGF = platelet-derived growth factor; PDL-CTX = peptide isolated from young cultures of periodontal ligament cells.
[‡]These are primary cultures obtained from young individuals (less than 20 years of age).
[§]These are either new primary cultures obtained from older individuals (greater than 70 years of age) or young periodontal ligament cells that have become senescent in vitro.
[¶]See Table 10-3 for description.

population is more responsive to PDL-CTX than the parent population of periodontal ligament cells. This observation suggests the possibility that PDL-CTX may be secreted by one subpopulation of periodontal ligament cells with a maximum response observed by a different subpopulation. Thus, this factor may have both autocrine and paracrine effects on the heterogeneous periodontal ligament cell population.

# Periodontal cell biology and oncogenes

Current studies in several laboratories are investigating the role of proto-oncogenes as critical determinants in normal cell function (Otto et al 1981; Piwnica-Worms et al 1987; Ralston and Bishop 1985). *Ets 1* expression has been demonstrated to be elevated in chicken cells of mesodermal lineage during development of small blood vessels. Barbacid and Parada (1986) have shown that *Trk*, in the mouse system, is limited to specific parts of the peripheral nervous system. Recently a variant of the *src* gene product, pp60[c-src(+)], has been shown to play a critical role in adult nerve cell function. Most, if not all, of the effect of oncogene expression (biologically active peptides) resides in signal transduction. There is now a substantial amount of data that indicate that phosphorylation of specific sites on kinases controls much of the observed activity. Phosphorylation can either activate or suppress the activity of a kinase (Warren and Nelson 1987). For example, the *src* product is not normally present or is present at low levels in most cells, except for blood platelets and neurons, which contain high levels. In the quiescent cell, extensive phosphorylation on tyrosine suppresses the kinase activity. Phosphorylation in the amino-terminal region, which occurs on serine and threonine during mitosis, appears to activate the enzyme. It has been suggested that because pp60[c-src] is phosphorylated and activated just before mitosis in NIH 3T3 cells, and is deactivated and dephosphorylated near the end of cell division, it might help regulate mitosis (Chackalaparampil and

Shalloway 1988). Several studies have indicated that both purified maturation-promoting factor (MPF), a well-known cell cycle regulator, and p34$^{cdc2}$, a catalytic component of MPF, can phosphorylate pp60$^{c\text{-}src}$ at the serine and threonine residues. These studies further suggest that pp60$^{c\text{-}src}$ may be involved in the regulation of certain mitotic events such as the changes in cell morphology that occur just before cell division. Cdc2 is a protein kinase. The fact that p34$^{cdc2}$ phosphorylates pp60$^{c\text{-}src}$ suggests that the c-*src* product, usually considered an upstream relay for messages sent from the cell membrane to the nucleus, is also regulated by cell cycle controls on its kinase activity that help control the rate of cell division. Other studies have shown that as cells enter mitosis, cdc2 dephosphorylation and p34 activation must occur before mitosis can continue (Nüsse and Egner 1984). Additional findings have shown that the c-*mos* enzyme, pp39$^{mos}$, is a proximal effector of meiosis. It is required to activate a precursor to MPF, pre-MPF, known to exist in premature oocytes in an inactive form. This review of recent important discoveries points out the level of complexity associated with cell replication. Cell replication is an essential event for tissue regeneration. In the periodontal research community, no investigation has been done on periodontal ligament cell replication at the molecular level.

The existence of more than 50 oncogenes has prompted a classification of oncogenes based on their shared functional properties. One of the classifications that has been accepted categorizes oncogenes on the basis of nuclear or cytoplasmic localization of function. Some of the nuclear oncogenes of interest are cellular genes that exhibit some structural homology with each other, specifically *myc*, N-*myc*, *myb*, and *E1A*. Experimentally, one of the most readily measured attributes of this group of oncogenes is their ability to convert a pri-

mary tissue culture cell, of limited replicative potential, into a cell that can be passaged in culture without restrictions. These experiments (commonly referred to as *transfection studies*) establish an immortalized cell line. Other phenotypic changes can also be associated with immortalization. For example, recent studies have indicated that transfection of human embryo fibroblasts, with the human c-*myc* oncogene, allows the fibroblasts to grow at lower serum concentrations and at significantly lower cell density in monolayer culture.

DNA-mediated (transfection) gene transfer experiments were used to show that the c-*myc* product is an intracellular messenger of the PDGF mitogenic signal. More recently, it has been demonstrated that microinjected c-*myc* protein induces DNA synthesis in quiescent 3T3 cells. This suggests that the c-*myc* protein is an intracellular competence signal, while PDGF initiates its competence signal only by a receptor-mediated event. It is also possible that the c-*myc* protein acts in concert with the other PDGF-inducible gene products to mediate competence in a variety of cell types. The other highly characterized PDGF-inducible gene is c-*fos*. Both genes are nuclear, DNA-binding, low-abundance, high-turnover phosphoproteins. They appear to function as regulatory peptides for gene expression, turning on or off whole sets of genes. Constitutive expression of the c-*myc* gene could be common in c-*myc*-transfected cells because this type of deregulation could lead to immortalization.

Present investigations in our laboratory have indicated that PDGF is one of the primary mitogenic signals for freshly cultured periodontal ligament cells (see Table 10-3). Regardless of in vivo age origin, all of our primary cultures lose responsiveness and then fail to respond to either PDGF or bFGF after 25 to 50 cumulative population doublings. Generally this type of response is similar for all primary human cell cultures. Other laboratories are studying the effect of various growth factors on primary cultures of periodontal ligament cells and gingival fibroblasts. Thus, depending on the passage number of the primary culture, it is possible to obtain different results. This in effect would make comparisons of periodontal ligament cell data between laboratories very difficult if not impossible.

The goal of this laboratory's transfection experiments was to develop an immortalized periodontal ligament cell line that would phenotypically resemble freshly cultured young periodontal ligament cells. The data suggest that the human c-*myc*-transfected cell line, PDL-L1, responds to various growth factors in a manner similar to that of primary cultures of young periodontal ligament cells (Figs 10-1 to 10-5).

# Periodontal regeneration and biology of aging

Biologic aging of tissues is a phenomenon that has so far eluded all efforts to determine its etiology. Numerous theories have been proposed to account for tissue changes categorized as "age-related," but none have received general acceptance by scientists involved in the study of aging. Despite the absence of an accepted theory, recent progress has been made in our understanding of the tissue and organ changes associated with aging (Sokal 1985).

Morphologic changes related to aging are relatively well defined. Decreased cellularity of tissues is visible at the light microscopic level, while other changes may be seen only by electron microscopy. The generally accepted observations are decreased cellular activity as evidenced by hyalinization of stromal tissues and vacuolization and loss of cellular organelles. These occurrences could be attributed to a loss of vascularity with a resulting decrease in available growth factor or reduced signal

transduction or reduced expression of specific oncogenes or increased expression of specific repressor oncogenes (Hall 1976).

Connective tissue matrix changes in aging have initiated much interest for more than 20 years and appear to vary according to the tissues studied. Collagen appears, in some instances, to undergo such great degenerative changes with age that it may be difficult to differentiate it from elastin by histochemical methods. Sex differences in the amount of collagen in normal adults are well documented; men have more skin collagen and lose it at a slower rate than do women. Apparent age-related changes in the structure of matrix proteins such as elastin have also been documented. It is well documented that adult periodontitis increases in prevalence and severity with increasing age. The exact mechanism of this increase is not known (Hall 1976).

On the molecular level, age-related alterations in the primary structure of both elastin and collagen have been determined. Changes in cross-linking of collagen and amounts of chondroitin sulfate may also signify tissue aging. Changes in amounts and biologic activity of some serum enzymes and other proteins with advanced age and altered hormonal states have also been noted, although the significance of most of these changes is as yet undetermined (Hall 1976; Kanuzo 1980). Receptor changes in aging may also be significant, suggesting decreased signal transduction or decreased oncogene expression. Changes in oncogene expression are just beginning to f e examined. Because there are presently no molecular biology studies of the periodontal support apparatus, it is difficult to project which oncogenes are important for periodontal ligament cell function.

When we examined primary periodontal ligament cell cultures from donors of different ages, we observed an age-dependent relationship to function. That is, cells obtained from younger donors (below the age of 20 years) phenotypically behave differently than do cells obtained from aged individuals (above the age of 70 years). Both sets of cultures were initiated and passaged at identical times so that in vitro senescence was avoided. A second observation was that primary cultures passaged to senescence in vitro resembled an old cell phenotype. These observations are noted in the motility and proliferation studies with PDGF, bFGF, and TGF-$\beta$ used as chemoattractants or mitogens (Figs 10-1 to 10-5). In all of these studies, the "young cells" represent a responsive population to adhesion, migration, and proliferation, whereas the "old cells" represent a refractive population.

## Significance and future directions

The overall significance and association of these specific topics (with respect to periodontal regeneration) resides in the observation that young periodontal ligament cells (in vitro or in vivo) have the ability to remain in a "repair phenotype" (ie, are able to repair a defect even in the presence of a bacterial insult), whereas old periodontal ligament cells express a "maintenance phenotype" (ie, are only able to maintain tissue integrity without bacterial insult). We have demonstrated that periodontal ligament cells have a decreased response to stimulation by b-FGF, PDGF, and TGF-$\beta$ as they age (either new primary cultures from older donors or old primary cultures from younger donors). This decreased response is observed in reduced chemotactic behavior and reduced ability to incorporate $^3$H-TdR into DNA (see Table 10-4). Part of the mechanism of periodontal disease progression, increasing with age, may be the periodontal ligament cells' inability to maintain a repair phenotype. Transfection of young primary cultures of periodontal ligament cells from young donors, by insertion of c-*myc*, results in a population of periodontal ligament cells that maintains the young (or repair) phenotype in culture.

The role of oncogenes in periodontal ligament cell function has not been examined. We have observed that c-*myc* can confer an immortalization on primary periodontal ligament cell cultures. These transfected cells require reduced amounts of all matrix and growth factors for proliferation. One of the gene products of the c-*sis* oncogene is a molecule with a large degree of homology to PDGF. Thus, we also maintain that the repair phenotype (young cells) is determined by high expression of specific oncogenes, which could include c-*myc* and c-*sis*.

A peptide isolated from young cultures of periodontal ligament cells, termed *PDL-CTX*, is a potent chemotactic and mitogenic signal for all periodontal ligament cells. Exposure of young periodontal ligament cells to PDL-CTX amplifies the effect of both b-FGF and PDGF on these cells. Old periodontal ligament cells can be induced to exhibit increased responsiveness to b-FGF and PDGF by exposure to PDL-CTX. This study suggests that the maintenance phenotype or cells with increasing senescence may be modulated by PDL-CTX. During the aging process we project that a decreased concentration of available PDL-CTX results in an "at-risk" tissue, which would be consistent with increased prevalence of periodontal tissue destruction with increasing age. Because the aged cells present with a refractive phenotype to previously identified growth factors, exogenous application of PDL-CTX may induce a responsive phenotype. Thus, a repair phenotype would be created. These anticipated results have been confirmed in limited in vivo studies independent to this laboratory. Present studies reside in building a PDL-CTX gene as defined by the amino acid sequence. With the current technology advancing at such a rapid rate, we project that the future of reparative periodontal regeneration resides with the possibility of gene correction, gene amplification, or gene replacement therapy.

## Acknowledgments

Supported in part by V.A. Merit Review grant 6577-010 and USPHS Grants DE08188, DE09411, DE09219; and in part by CYTOTAXIS, Inc.

## References

Akers RM, Mosher DF, Lilian J. Promotion of retinal neurite outgrowth by substratum bound fibronectin. *Dev Biol* 1981;86:179–188.

Assoian RK, Grothendorst GR, Miller DM, Sporn MB. Cellular transformation by coordinated action of three polypeptide growth factors from human platelets. *Nature* 1984;309:804–806.

Assoian RK, Sporn MB. Transforming growth factor in human platelets: release during platelet degranulation and action on vascular smooth muscle cells. *J Cell Biol* 1986;102:1217–1223.

Azizkhan RG, Azizkhan JC, Zetter BR, Folkman J. Mast cell heparin stimulates migration of capillary endothelial cells in vitro. *J Exp Med* 1980;152:931–944.

Barbacid M, Parada LF. Human oncogenes. *Imp Adv Oncol* 1986;3:3–22.

Bowen-Pope DF, Seifert RA. Exogenous and endogenous sources of PDGF-like molecules and their potential roles in vascular biology. In: *Cancer Cells.* Cold Spring Harbor, NY: Cold Spring Harbor Press; 1985:183–188.

Chackalaparampil I, Shalloway D. Altered phosphorylation and activation of pp60src. *Cell* 1988;52:801.

Deuel TF, Kimura A, Machana S, Tong BD. Platelet derived growth factor: roles in normal and V-*sis* transformed cells. *Cancer Surveys* 1985;4:633–653.

Gaus-Muller A, Kleinman HK, Martin GR, Schiffmann E. Role of attachment factors and attractants in fibroblast chemotaxis. *J Lab Clin Med* 1980;96:1071–1080.

Grotendorst GR, Seppa HE, Kleinman HK, Martin GR. Attachment of smooth muscle cells to collagen and their migration towards platelet derived growth factor. *Proc Natl Acad Sci USA* 1981;78:3669–3672.

Hall DA. *The Aging of Connective Tissue.* New York: Academic Press, 1976.

Kanuzo MS. *Biochemistry of Aging.* London: Academic Press, 1980.

Kehrl JH, Wakefield LM, Roberts AB, et al. Production of transforming growth factor ß by human T-lymphocytes and its potential role in the regulation of T cell growth. *J Cell Growth* 1986;163:1037–1050.

Liotta LA,. Mandler R, Murano G, et al. Tumor cell autocrine motility factor. *Proc Natl Acad Sci USA* 1986;83:3302–3306.

Loesche WJ. The bacterial etiology of dental decay and periodontal disease: the specific plaque hypothesis. *Clin Dent* 1982;2:1–54.

McCarthy JB, Palm SL, Furcht LT. Migration by haptotaxis of a Schwann cell tumor line to the basement membrane glycoprotein laminin. *J Cell Biol* 1983;97:772–777.

McCarthy JB, Furcht LT. Laminin and fibronectin promote the haptotactic migration of B16 mouse melanoma cells in vitro. *J Cell Biol* 1984;98:1474–1480.

Mehlman T, Maciag T. The interaction of endothelial cell growth factor with heparin: characterization by receptor and antibody recognition. *Proc Natl Acad Sci USA* 1985;82:6138–6143.

Nüsse M, Egner HJ. Can Nocodazole, an inhibitor of microtubule formation, be used to synchronize mammalian cells? *Cell Tissue Kinet* 1984;17:13–23.

Otto AM, Ulrich MO, Zumbe A, Jimenez de Asna L. Microtubule disrupting agents affect two different events regulating the initiation of DNA synthesis in Swiss 3T3 cells. *Proc Natl Acad Sci USA* 1981;78:3063.

Piwnica-Worms H, Saunders KB, Roberts TM, Smith AE, Cheng SH. Tyrosine phosphorylation regulates the biochemical and biological properties of pp60src. *Cell* 1987;49:75.

Ralston R, Bishop JM. The product of the proto-oncogene c-*src* is modified during the cellular response to PDGF. *Proc Natl Acad Sci USA* 1985;82:7845.

Ross R, Rainer EW, Bowen-Pope DF. The biology of platelet-derived growth factor. *Cell* 1986;46:155–169.

Schiffmann E, Gallin JE. Biochemistry of phagocyte chemotaxis. In: Horecker BL, Stadtman ER, eds. *Current Topics in Cellular Regulation.* New York: Academic Press, 1979;15:203–216.

Selvig KA. Current concepts of connective tissue attachment to diseased tooth surfaces. *J Biol Buccale* 1983;11:79–94.

Seppa HE, Grotendorst GR, Seppa ST, Schiffmann E, Martin GR. Platelet derived growth factor is chemotactic for fibroblasts. *J Cell Biol* 1982;92:584–588.

Seyedin SM, Thompson AY, Bentz H, et al. Cartilage-inducing factor-A, apparent identity to transforming growth factor ß. *J Biol Chem* 1986;261:5693–5695.

Sokal RS. *Molecular Biology of Aging: Gene Stability and Gene Expression.* New York: Raven Press, 1985.

Sporn MB, Roberts AB. Peptide growth factors and inflammation, tissue repair and cancer. *J Clin Invest* 1986;78:329–332.

Tanner ACR, Haffer C, Bratthal GT, Visconti RA, Socransky SS. A study of the bacteria associated with the advancing periodontitis in man. *J Clin Periodontol* 1979;6:278–289.

Terranova VP, DiFlorio R, Lyall RM, Hic S, Friesel R, Maciag T. Human endothelial cells are chemotactic to endothelial cell growth factor and heparin. *J Cell Biol* 1985;101:2330–2334.

Terranova VP, Lyall RM. Chemotaxis of human gingival epithelial cells to laminin: a mechanism for epithelial cell apical migration. *J Periodontol* 1986; 57:311–317.

Terranova VP, Franzetti LC, Hic S, et al. A biochemical approach to periodontal regeneration: tetracycline treatment of dentin promotes fibroblast adhesion and growth. *J Periodont Res* 1986;21:301–337.

Terranova VP, Hic S, Franzetti L, Lyall RM, Wikesjö UME. A biochemical approach to periodontal regeneration. AFSCM: assays for specific cell migration. *J Periodontol* 1987;58:247–257.

Terranova VP, Wikesjö UME. Extracellular matrices and polypeptide growth factors as mediators of functions of cells of the periodontium: a review. *J Periodontol* 1988a;58:371–380.

Terranova VP, Wikesjö UME. Chemotaxis of human periodontal ligament cells to various biological response modifiers. *Adv Dent Res* 1988b;2:215–222.

Warren SL, Nelson WJ. Nonmitogenic morphoregulatory action of pp60v-src on multicellular epithelial structures. *Mol Cell Biol* 1987;7:1326–1337.

# Chapter 11

# The Role of Growth Factors in Periodontal Repair and Regeneration

Samuel E. Lynch

For efficient tissue repair to be achieved, cells from around a wound must proliferate, migrate into the wounded area, and, once within the wound, lay down extracellular matrix. As a result of this process, the tissue void created by the wounding insult fills up with new cells and their surrounding matrix. For tissue regeneration to be achieved, the cells that occupy the wound must be of the same type and oriented in the same pattern as the cells that originally occupied that space. In addition, the extracellular matrix produced by those cells must be of the same type and orientation and must form the same structures as those that were present before the insult occurred. To achieve repair, structural, but not necessarily functional, integrity must be restored.

The pathogenesis, and therefore regeneration/repair, of periodontal lesions is perhaps one of the most complex to occur in the body. At least six tissue types are involved in the repair of a periodontal lesion: the gingival epithelium, gingival connective tissue, periodontal ligament, tooth root surface cementum, alveolar bone, and all the corresponding vasculature. Nowhere else in the body are epithelium and mineralized and nonmineralized connective tissues juxtaposed in such proximity. For regeneration of the periodontium to occur, all of these components must be restored to their original position and architecture. Thus the cells that form these tissues must repopulate a wound site and produce the appropriate matrix.

Barrier membranes facilitate periodontal regeneration by allowing only cells from the tissues originally present to repopulate the root surface following surgical therapy. However, such barriers do not promote the cellular processes necessary for repair or regeneration (ie, proliferation, migration, and matrix synthesis) (Aukhil and Iglhaut 1988). How does the body promote these processes so essential to all tissue repair and regeneration? Our current understanding leads us to believe that polypeptide growth factors are key regulators of these processes.

*Growth factors* is a general term used to denote a class of naturally occurring proteins that function in the body to promote the mitogenesis (proliferation), directed migration, and metabolic activity of cells. Thus, the three key cellular events in tissue repair are mitogenesis, migration, and matrix synthesis and remodelling ($M^3$). Numerous growth factors have been isolated from tissues and characterized; the principal growth factors used to promote

179

wound healing are shown in Table 11-1. We now know that growth factors are cell specific, meaning that a particular growth factor acts only on defined cell types. For example, keratinocyte growth factor (KGF) will stimulate epithelial cells but not fibroblasts or endothelial cells, while fibroblast growth factor (FGF) will stimulate several cell types, including fibroblasts and endothelial cells.

For a growth factor to mediate repair of the periodontium, it need only affect the tissues necessary for wound closure, ie, the fibrous connective tissue and epithelium. However, for a growth factor to affect periodontal regeneration, it must be able to stimulate formation of mineralized as well as nonmineralized tissues. A combination of growth factors may more effectively stimulate these diverse processes of regeneration than any single growth factor. A combination might consist of one factor that promotes mineralized tissue (bone and cementum) formation, and another factor that stimulates formation of the nonmineralized connective tissues, ie, periodontal ligament and gingival connective tissue. As will be described subsequently, the latter approach using a combination of growth factors has been used successfully to enhance periodontal regeneration in beagle dogs with natural periodontal disease and nonhuman primates with ligature-induced disease (Lynch et al 1989a, 1991; Giannobile et al 1994; Rutherford et al 1992).

This chapter describes how the body naturally uses growth factors to heal nonmineralized and mineralized tissue wounds, the actions of the best-characterized growth factors, and how certain of these factors have been used to promote periodontal regeneration. Because periodontal regeneration requires the restoration of nonmineralized and mineralized tissues, the role of growth factors in the repair of each of these tissues will be discussed.

# The role of growth factors in wound repair

## Nonmineralized tissues

An injury involving subepithelial tissue results in disruption of the vascular supply in the area and subsequently in hemorrhage. Platelets initiate hemostasis by forming a cellular plug. In addition, fibrin, fibrinogen, and fibronectin are deposited to form a clot at the sites where the blood vessels are disrupted. Adhesion of platelets to the subendothelial tissues and their activation results in release of a variety of substances that accentuate the repair processes, the most potent of which appear to be polypeptide growth factors. Nearly equal amounts of platelet-derived growth factor (PDGF) and transforming growth factor beta (TGF-$\beta$) as well as proteins resembling epidermal growth factor (EGF) and transforming growth factor alpha (TGF-$\alpha$) are liberated following platelet activation (Assoian et al 1984). Once these growth factors have been deposited at the site of injury by platelets, they can initiate the repair process. Both PDGF and TGF-$\beta$ stimulate the influx of neutrophils into the wound site. The neutrophils act as the initial "clean-up crew" following injury by phagocytizing and digesting damaged tissue and bacteria. The TGF-$\beta$ also stimulates the influx of monocytes and macrophages into the wounded area. Usually these cells arrive somewhat after the neutrophils and continue to debride the area in preparation for the ingrowth of new tissue. Thus, growth factors can initiate inflammatory cell influx, the first stage of tissue repair.

The growth factors released from platelets can also stimulate the ingrowth of highly vascularized new connective tissue (termed *granulation tissue*). Granulation tissue formation results from macrophages, fibroblasts, and blood vessels that migrate

Table 11-1    Sources of growth factors at wound sites

| Growth factor | Major sources at the wound site |
|---|---|
| PDGF* | Platelets, macrophages, epithelial cells, endothelial cells,[†] smooth muscle cells, bone matrix |
| TGF-β* | Platelets, macrophages, activated T lymphocytes,[†] osteoblasts, immature chondrocytes, bone matrix |
| EGF/TGF-α | Platelets, macrophages, epithelial cells, eosinophils |
| IGF-1* | Plasma, epithelial cells, endothelial cells,[†] fibroblasts,[†] smooth muscle cells,[†] osteoblasts, bone matrix |
| bFGF | Macrophages, endothelial cells,[†] osteoblasts, immature and mature chondrocytes, bone matrix |

*For the purpose of this review PDGF-AA, AB, and BB will simply be designated as PDGF, and TGF-β1 and β2 will be designated as TGF-β. IGF-2 (skeletal growth factor) is also produced by osteoblasts and is present in bone matrix.
[†]Hypothesized from in vitro experiments.

into the wound with similar kinetics. Macrophages themselves produce a multitude of growth factors. It appears likely that growth factors from macrophages are responsible for the continued stimulation of the surrounding cells because platelets provide only the initial deposition of growth factors during clotting. Other cells surrounding the wound also produce growth factors in a strikingly well-controlled manner. For example, epithelial cells in normal skin neither make nor are responsive to PDGF. However, as little as 1 day after cutaneous injury, and peaking at 3 days after injury, epithelial cells produce large amounts of PDGF (Antoniades et al 1991, 1993). The level of PDGF production then decreases and is present in only very low levels at the time when re-epithelialization has been completed. Other growth factors are also produced by epithelial cells and other cell types following injury. Table 11-1 lists the sources of the most well-characterized growth factors at the site of injury involving epithelium, underlying connective tissue, or bone.

Neovascularization (the biologic process of restoring the blood supply to the new tissue within the wound) is also stimulated by several growth factors. Among the most potent angiogenic factors are bFGF and aFGF (basic and acidic fibroblast growth factors), as well as TGF-α and TGF-β. Both bFGF and aFGF act directly on endothelial cells to stimulate their proliferation, and aFGF in particular stimulates tubule formation (Gospodarowicz et al 1987). The TGF-β most likely enhances angiogenesis indirectly by increasing the influx of macrophages, which in turn produce a variety of angiogenic substances.

Components of fibroplasia, which includes the influx and proliferation of fibroblasts and the deposition of fibronectin, glycosaminoglycans (making up the provisional extracellular matrix), and collagens are stimulated by most growth factors. Table 11-2 summarizes the effects of the best-characterized growth factors on connective tissue repair. The most potent stimulator of fibronectin and collagen production is TGF-β, while in most circumstances FGF decreases collagen production by fibroblasts. Platelet-derived growth factor and FGF both enhance the influx of fibroblasts into a wound site and increase provisional extracellular matrix production. Platelet-derived growth factor in combination with insulinlike growth factor (IGF-1) stimulates recruitment and proliferation of fibroblasts and increased collagen synthesis and maturity.

Table 11-2    Effects of growth factors on connective tissue repair

| Activity | Growth factor | | | |
|---|---|---|---|---|
|  | PDGF | TGF-β | bFGF | PDGF+IGF-1 |
| Fibroblast influx | ++ | 0 | + | ++ |
| Fibroblast proliferation | + | +/— | + | ++ |
| Fibronectin synthesis | 0 | ++ | + | ? |
| Glycosaminoglycan synthesis | ++ | 0 | ++ | ++ |
| Collagen synthesis | + | +++ | — | +++ |
| Collagen maturation | 0 | ++ | — | ++ |
| Collagenase activity | ++ | — | ++ | ? |
| Myofibroblast generation | + | — | 0 | ? |
| Endothelial cell migration | 0 | 0 | ++ | ? |
| Macrophage influx | 0 | + | 0 | 0 |

+ Marginally increased; ++ Increased; +++ Substantially increased; — Decreased; 0 No effect; ? Not determined.

Growth factors also affect the rate of re-epithelialization of a wound. While EGF and TGF-α directly increase the rate of re-epithelialization, bFGF and PDGF may enhance re-epithelialization indirectly in impaired skin wound healing models by stimulating a healthy bed of new connective tissue, but neither appears to accelerate re-epithelialization of skin wounds in healthy animals (Lynch et al 1989b; Greenhalgh et al 1990). The effects of TGF-β are dose and time dependent. In general, it inhibits epithelial cell proliferation but appears to stimulate migration of these cells.

The mechanism by which TGF-β affects this dual response on epithelial cells is not fully understood. However, it may be that the increased epithelial cell migration is caused by the enhanced production of fibronectin, which TGF-β stimulates. Although epithelial cells in normal intact skin do not express receptors for fibronectin (ie, they do not bind fibronectin), the epithelial cells in a wound do express receptors and bind fibronectin. *In fact, epithelial cells are attracted to proteolytic fragments of fibronectin and even secrete fibronectin themselves when moving over a wound.* Interestingly, laminin, once thought to be important for epithelial cell migration, has been shown to be a poor substrate for epithelial cell movement (Donaldson and Mahan 1984). In direct comparisons, it has been found that basal keratinocytes will migrate when apposed to fibronectin and types I and IV collagens, but that migration of these cells is inhibited when apposed to laminin (Woodley et al 1990). These data clearly call into question the use of fibronectin to promote connective tissue attachment following periodontal surgery.

The interactions of growth factors in nonmineralized tissue repair are illustrated in Fig 11-1. These interactions have been more extensively reviewed elsewhere (Kiritsy and Lynch 1993; Lynch 1990). Clearly, the healing of nonmineralized tissues by themselves involves a complex series of cell-cell and cell-macromolecular interactions. Although these interactions have been primarily described in skin wounds, similar processes are no doubt involved in the healing of soft tissues of the periodontium following acute injury. In fact, the principles described above have thus far been found to universally apply to the healing of external wounds of nearly all adult mammals.

The topical addition of exogenous growth factors can accelerate many of the components of soft tissue healing (Table 11-3). As summarized in the preceding discussion

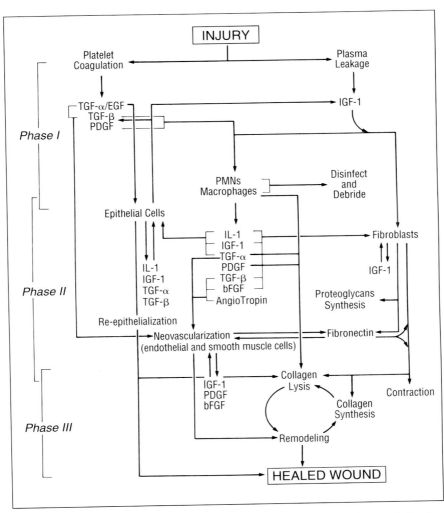

Fig 11-1   Proposed interactions of natural endogenous growth factors following injury to epithelium and underlying connective tissues based on in vitro and in vivo experimental observations. (From Lynch 1990 and Kiritsy and Lynch 1993; used with permission.)

and tables, which components are affected depends on which growth factors are applied. Of the nonmineralized tissues of the periodontium, the regeneration of the periodontal ligament is the most problematic. The periodontal ligament is composed, at least in part, of fibroblasts, blood vessels, and collagen. To achieve its restoration fol-lowing periodontal disease, we must promote its coronal establishment. Thus, growth factors that promote fibroblast prolif-eration and migration as well as collagen synthesis appear to be good candidates for enhancing new periodontal ligament forma-tion (although for a true new periodontal lig-ament to form there must also be new

Table 11-3   Vulnerary influence of growth factors on the major biologic processes required for soft tissue repair (adapted from Pierce 1991)

| Growth factor | Re-epithelialization | Neovessel formation | Provisional extracellular matrix | Collagen |
|---|---|---|---|---|
| PDGF | 0/+* | + | + | + |
| TGF-β | +§/— | ++ | 0/+¶ | +++ |
| EGF/TGF-α | ++ | 0/+ | 0 | 0 |
| IGF-1 | 0 | 0 | 0 | 0 |
| bFGF | + | ++ | ++ | 0 |
| PDGF+IGF-1 | ++ | ++ | ++ | — |
| PDGF+TGF-α | + | + | ++ | ++ |

*Secondary to increased extracellular matrix and collagen production in impaired wound healing models.
§The effects of TGF-β1 on epithelialization appear to be dose and time dependent. It may increase re-epithelialization secondary to increased granulation tissue production and epithelial cell migration, but its direct effect on epithelial proliferation is inhibitory.
¶Primarily fibronectin.
+ Marginally increased; ++ Increased; +++ Substantially increased; — Decreased; 0 No effect.

cementum and new bone formation, a problem to be discussed shortly). Of the most well-characterized growth factors, PDGF and IGF-1 are the most potent chemoattractants for fibroblasts, including those derived from the periodontal ligament (Matsuda et al 1991) (Table 11-4). Terranova and coworkers (1987) have also demonstrated the potent chemotactic nature of aFGF on fibroblasts derived from periodontal ligament tissues. They have found that aFGF is 10,000 times more potent in inducing directed fibroblast migration than fibronectin. Both PDGF and FGF can also promote periodontal ligament fibroblast proliferation. No amount of fibronectin can stimulate the proliferation of fibroblasts to the extent achieved with nanogram amounts of PDGF or FGF. The combination of PDGF and IGF-1 promotes greater proliferation of periodontal ligament fibroblasts than PDGF alone (Matsuda et al 1991; Lynch unpublished observation). In general, TGF-β appears to promote more significant deposition of fibroblast collagen than any of the other individual growth factors (Lynch et al 1989b). However, TGF-β is not chemotactic for fibroblasts, and its ability to stimulate fibroblast proliferation appears to be highly

dependent on dose and the local environment. The combination of PDGF and IGF-1 has also been shown to promote collagen deposition equal to that achieved using TGF-β (Lynch et al 1989b). It has been reported that EGF and TGF-α increase collagen production only if given at high doses for prolonged periods, and at these doses both EGF and TGF-α increase the rate of re-epithelialization, an event detrimental to periodontal regeneration. (Buckley et al 1985; Schultz et al 1987).

**Mineralized tissues**

Less is currently known about the role of endogenous growth factors or the effects of exogenously applied growth factors in the repair of bone wounds. As is the case with wounded nonmineralized tissues, growth factors may be delivered to bone wounds by two routes: (1) from the vasculature via platelets and plasma, and (2) through local production by cells at the injured site. Thus, PDGF and TGF-β have been detected in the early hematoma following fracture healing. TGF-β, aFGF, and bFGF are produced locally adjacent to long bone fractures (Joyce et al 1990a). Moderate levels of

Table 11-4    Effects of growth factors on periodontal ligament cells* (from Lynch & Giannobile 1994)

| Growth factor | Mitogenesis | Migration | Metabolism** |
|---|---|---|---|
| PDGF | ++ | ++ | + |
| IGF-1 | + | ++ | + |
| FGF | ++ | ++ | − |
| TGF-ß | − | 0 | + |
| EGF | + | 0 | 0 |
| PDGF/IGF | +++ | +++ | ++ |
| TGF-ß/EGF | − | 0 | ? |

*Information derived from Matsuda et al, Terranova et al, and Lynch et al (Unpublished observations).
**As assessed by either total protein or collagen content.
− Inhibitory effect; 0 No effect; + Slight effect; ++ Moderate effect; +++ Strong effect.

Table 11-5    Effects of growth factors on bone formation and resorption

| Growth factor | Matrix synthesis | | Matrix degradation or bone resorption | Osteoblast influx |
|---|---|---|---|---|
| | Direct effect | Secondary to mitogenesis | | |
| aFGF | — | + | 0 | ? |
| bFGF | — | + | 0 | ? |
| PDGF | +/0 | + | + | + |
| TGF-ß | +/—* | +/—* | +/—* | + |
| IGF-1 | + | + | — | ? |
| PDGF+IGF-1 | + | ++ | — | ? |
| TGF-ß+IGF-1 | ? | ++ | ? | + |
| PDGF+IGF-1+TGF-ß | ? | +++ | ? | + |

+ Increased; — Decreased; 0 No effect; ? Not determined; * Dose- and local environment–dependent.

PDGF gene expression are also present in the fracture callus. Both TFG-ß and the FGFs are produced in areas of cartilage and bone formation in the healing of the long bone fracture. Interestingly, PDGF is a more potent stimulator of cellular proliferation within the fracture callus than either TGF-ß or bFGF; PDGF also increases collagen gene expression when added to the fracture callus (Joyce et al 1990a). Subperiosteal injections of TGF-ß into the newborn rat femur resulted in extensive cartilage formation and osteoclast-mediated resorption of the cortical bone. The cartilage mass was replaced with bone after the daily injections were stopped (Joyce et al 1990a, 1990b). In the same model system, injections of PDGF resulted in intramembranous bone formation, that is, bone formation in the absence of cartilage (Joyce et al 1990a).

Alveolar bone formation occurs by the intramembranous route as does bone formation in the calvariae. Numerous studies have been performed in vitro to determine the effects of growth factors on bone formation in the fetal rat calvaria. The findings from these studies are summarized in Table 11-5 (Canalis et al 1989a). The growth factors aFGF, bFGF, and PDGF increase a cell population of the osteoblast lineage capable of synthesizing collagen but do not directly increase collagen production by differentiated osteoblasts. Both TGF-ß and IGF-1 can increase the proliferation of osteoblasts (or their precursors) and collagen production by differentiated osteoblasts. Both PDGF and TGF-β are also capable of stimulating bone resorption (Cochran et al 1991; Tashjian et al 1985). The effects of TGF-β in particular appear to be highly dependent on the dose and local environment, because it has also been reported to inhibit osteoblast proliferation, bone formation, and stimulate formation of osteoclastlike cells (Antosz et al 1989; Chenu et al 1988). The combination of PDGF and IGF-1 increases bone matrix apposition in organ culture more than PDGF, IGF-1, or TGF-β individually (Pfeilschifter et al 1990; Lynch unpublished observations). Likewise, the combination of TGF-β and IGF-1 is more potent in stimulating matrix apposition than any individual growth factor (Pfeilschifter et al 1990). The addition of IGF-1 to PDGF counteracts the enhanced collagen degradation seen in vitro when PDGF is used alone (Canalis et al 1989b). Maximal proliferation of cultured adult human osteoblasts was seen with a combination of PDGF, IGF-1, TGF-β, and EGF (Piché and Graves 1989).

Studies of the chemotactic effects of growth factors on osteoblasts would be especially valuable to assess their effects on periodontal regeneration. The ability to enhance directed migration of osteoblasts is particularly important for periodontal regeneration because bone is often present only at the apical portion of the periodontal lesion. Thus, for complete regeneration to occur, the bone-forming cells must migrate coronally, often several millimeters. Without the presence of potent chemotactic agents, it does not appear that such coronal migration of adult human osteoblasts would occur, even in the presence of putative osteoconductive materials or barrier membranes. Recently, the effects of PDGF and TGF-β have been evaluated on osteoblast influx or migration. It was demonstrated that bone cells migrate in a dose-dependent manner toward an increasing gradient of PDGF or TGF-β (Gilardetti et al 1992; Pfeilshifter et al 1990).

## Which growth factors promote periodontal regeneration?

Given the preceding overview, the question remains: Which growth factors will promote regeneration of the periodontium? There is as yet no definitive answer to this question (except for the combination of PDGF and IGF-1, which will be discussed below). However, current knowledge suggests advantages and disadvantages to the use of certain growth factors and raises specific questions that need to be answered. Neither EGF nor TGF-α, at least by themselves, appears likely to enhance periodontal regeneration, because both promote bone resorption, are weak enhancers of connective tissue formation, and are strong stimulators of epithelial migration and proliferation. Both aFGF and bFGF will likely promote the coronal migration of periodontal ligament fibroblasts. Because coronal migration of periodontal ligament cells is thought to be a prerequisite for new attachment, this would suggest that the FGFs could promote regeneration; however, other studies indicate they may reduce collagen production by fibroblasts while inducing collagenase synthesis. Whether this reduction in collagen is significant enough to affect periodontal ligament formation is not known. Both aFGF and bFGF are likely to promote proliferation of alveolar bone cells, but whether this would in turn lead to increased bone matrix formation is unclear since FGFs down regulate transcription of the type I collagen gene. Preliminary data evaluating the effects of a combination of TGF-β, bFGF, and IGF-2 indicated no enhancement of bone formation 4 weeks after application to surgically created defects in dogs (Selvig et al 1994). However, the dose may have been too low to effect a response.

The most potent individual growth factor for stimulating bone matrix apposition in culture is TGF-β; it thus would likely be a potent stimulus for alveolar bone formation. The fact that TGF-β is not chemotactic for periodontal ligament fibroblasts suggests that it alone will not promote the coronal migration of these cells, however. The net result of rapid bone growth in the absence of coronal migration of periodontal ligament cells could be ankylosis.

Platelet-derived growth factor is chemotactic for periodontal ligament osteoblasts and fibroblasts and thus will likely promote the coronal migration of periodontal ligament cells. In addition, in vitro data show that PDGF and IGF-1 promote fibroblast and osteoblast proliferation, collagen (especially IGF-1) and noncollagen (especially PDGF) protein synthesis, and bone matrix formation. Nearly all of these activities are increased even further when PDGF and IGF-1 are combined. The following findings suggest that the combination of PDGF and IGF-1 would enhance regeneration of all the components of the periodontium: (1) PDGF and IGF-1 are chemotactic and mitogenic for periodontal ligament fibroblasts; (2) PDGF is chemotactic for osteoblasts; (3) IGF-1 promotes collagenous protein synthesis and PDGF promotes primarily noncollagenous protein synthesis in bone cultures; (4) the combination of PDGF and IGF-1 promotes greater bone matrix formation than any individual growth factor; and (5) PDGF and IGF-1 interact synergistically to promote significant collagen formation and healing in soft tissue wounds.

# Effects of PDGF and IGF-1 on periodontal regeneration

A series of studies has been conducted to determine the effects of the combination of PDGF and IGF-1 (PDGF/IGF-1) on periodontal wound healing. These studies have ranged in duration from 2 weeks to 6 months and have examined the effects of PDGF/IGF-1 placed in a simple gel or incorporated into demineralized freeze-dried bone (DFDB) or beta tricalcium phosphate (TCP). So far these studies have been conducted primarily in older beagle dogs with natural periodontal disease and cynamologous primates with ligature-induced attachment loss.

On entry into the studies, all dogs exhibited natural, generalized severe gingivitis, bleeding on probing, large deposits of supragingival and subgingival plaque and calculus, 30% to 70% alveolar bone loss radiographically, and in most cases class III furcation defects. Two weeks after initial debridement, full-thickness periodontal flaps were elevated around all premolars. Granulation tissue was removed and the root surfaces were planed to remove all calculus and plaque deposits. The PDGF/IGF-1 was then applied topically to the bone and root surfaces. The gel containing the growth factors had previously been placed into a syringe, which made application around the teeth quick and easy. The DFDB and TCP with and without incorporated growth factors were applied from a sterile container using a small spatula and packed into the bone defects. The flaps were then sutured with their coronal margins adjacent to the cementoenamel junction.

Biopsy specimens were obtained at 2 weeks (gel/PDGF/IGF-1 or gel-only sites), 5, and 12 weeks (all treatments). Biopsies were also performed on a few gel/PDGF/IGF-1 or gel-only treated sites at 24 weeks to observe the histologic appearance of the new bone or periodontal ligament. Quantitative histometric analyses were performed on all 2-, 5-, and 12-week-old sites. Due to abscess formation and generalized extensive inflammation resulting from an absence of oral hygiene, only the 2- and 5-week sites could be statistically analyzed.

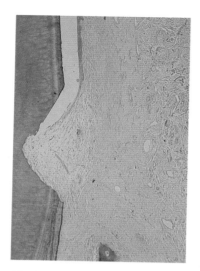

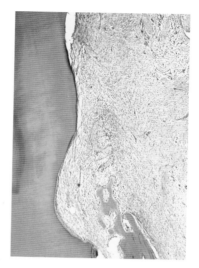

Fig 11-2a   Surgery plus placebo gel 2 weeks postoperatively. Specimen shows the alveolar crest and supracrestal connective tissue region. There is minimal evidence of osteogenic or cementogenic activity. Original magnification ×16.

Fig 11-2b   Surgery plus PDGF/IGF-1 2 weeks postoperatively. Specimen shows the alveolar crest and supracrestal connective tissue region. Abundant osteogenic and cementogenic activity is present. Original magnification ×16.

The results from these studies are summarized in Figs 11-2 to 11-8 (Lynch et al 1989a, 1991; Giannobile et al 1994). As seen in Figs 11-2 to 11-5, a consistent sequence of wound healing events was observed histologically. At 2 weeks the epithelium had migrated apically to the base of the instrumented root surface in the majority of control specimens receiving the gel alone. In areas of vertical bone defects, the epithelium was generally interposed between the crest of the nonsupporting alveolar bone and the root surface. There was almost no new cementum on the root surfaces. Dense randomly oriented collagen fibers occupied most of the area within infrabony defects 2 weeks postoperatively. In the supracrestal area of control specimens, no new bone formation was observed (Fig 11-2a). Near the base

of infrabony defects, small islands of new bone were present in proximity to the wall of the original bone defect.

In experimental specimens treated with PDGF/IGF-1, significant amounts of newly formed bone were present in both horizontal and vertical alveolar bone defects. At 2 weeks nearly all surfaces of the new bone were surrounded by a continuous layer of osteoblastlike cells (Fig 11-2b). The osteoblastlike cells present on the bone surface were often partially surrounded by new bone matrix, which suggests that active osteoid deposition was present at this time. Active bone formation was evident throughout the extent of new bone. The new bone became more immature as its distance from the original bone increased. An area of high cell density, or cellular "front," was often present within the con-

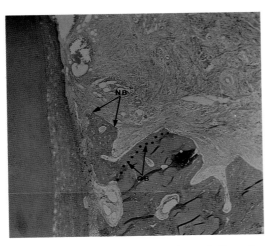

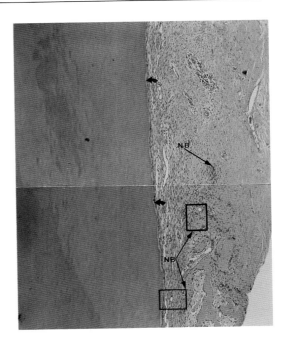

Fig 11-3a  Surgery plus placebo gel, 5 weeks postoperatively. The dotted line indicates the most coronal portion of the original bone (OB). A modest amount of new bone (NB) can be seen coronal to the old bone. There is no evidence of new cementum deposition along the surface of the root. Original magnification ×63.

Fig 11-3b  (Right) Surgery plus PDGF/IGF-1, 5 weeks postoperatively. New bone matrix (NB, straight arrows) is evident within the connective tissues adjacent to the root surface. The original bone is beyond the lower margin of the photomicrograph. An increase in cellularity (ie, a cellular "front") can be observed adjacent to the coronal portion of the new bone. In addition, the new bone is lined by a nearly continuous layer of osteoblasts. New cementum deposition on the tooth root surface is also evident (curved arrows). Original magnification ×63.

Fig 11-3c  Area outlined in the lower box of Fig 11-3b. New cementumlike deposits are seen on the root surface (straight arrows) as dense eosinophilic material on the outer aspect of the more purple root dentin. The new cementumlike material is lined by cells, some of which are partially or completely incorporated into the new cementum matrix. Large osteoblastlike cells are present adjacent to the bone matrix. The new cementum on the root surface and the new bone matrix are separated by the width of a healthy periodontium. Fibroblasts, blood vessels, and collagen bundles occupy the periodontal ligament space between the new cementum and new bone. Original magnification ×400.

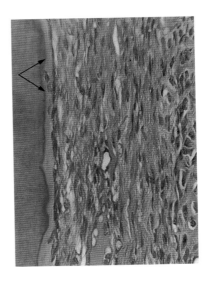

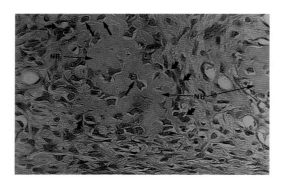

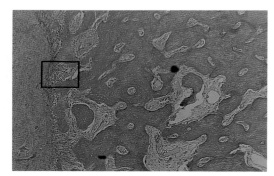

Fig 11-3d   Area outlined in the upper box of Fig 11-3b, showing islands of new bone matrix *(NB)*. Numerous osteoblasts are partially *(curved arrows)* or completely *(straight arrows)* surrounded by new bone matrix. Numerous mitotic figures are present. The phenotypic appearance of the osteoblasts is consistent with the presence of multiple stages of cell division. Numerous vessels are also evident. Original magnification ×400.

Fig 11-3e   PDGF/IGF-1–treated specimen, 5 weeks postoperatively, showing new bone growth in an area between the two roots of a premolar. This photomicrograph depicts the buccal surface of a new bone. No old bone is present within this field. The new bone contains numerous osteocytes, and its outer aspect is lined by a nearly continuous layer of osteoblasts. Areas of high cell density are present within the connective tissue immediately adjacent to the new osteoid. The cells in these areas are osteoblastic in appearance. Original magnification ×63.

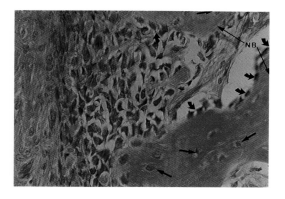

Fig 11-3f   Area outlined on Fig 11-3e. Numerous osteoblasts *(curved arrows)* are shown lining the new bone *(NB)*. Numerous osteocytes *(straight arrows)* completely surrounded by bone matrix are also present. Mitotic figures are present within many of the osteoblastlike cells within the connective tissue adjacent to the new bone, indicating these cells are undergoing active cell division. Original magnification ×400.

nective tissue immediately adjacent to the coronal extent of new osteoid. The cells within this area were osteoblastic in appearance. New bone was also seen on the periosteal surfaces of the original alveolar bone. New cementum was present on the root surface, having been deposited on both preexisting dentin and cementum. The new cementum was also often lined by a nearly continuous layer of cells.

At 5 weeks postoperatively (Figs 11-3a to f), the new bone was more dense in both control and treated sites than at 2 weeks. In PDGF/IGF-1–treated sites it was often still surrounded by osteoblasts. In fact, large clusters of osteoblastlike cells were seen adjacent to the new bone in treated sites (Figs 11-3d to f). In treated sites, the new cementum was still lined by a nearly continuous layer of cells (Fig

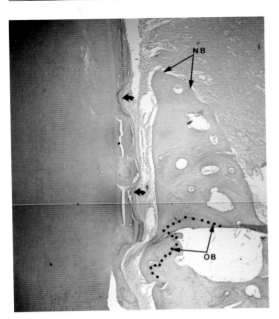

Fig 11-4a   Surgery plus placebo gel, 12 weeks postoperatively. The original alveolar crest *(OB)* is demarcated by the dotted line. A small amount of new bone *(NB)* and new cementum *(curved arrow)* is present coronal to the old bone. Original magnification ×63.

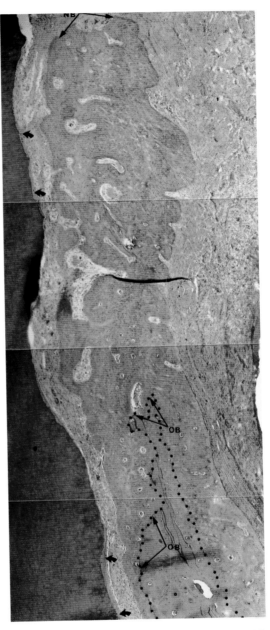

Fig 11-4b   Surgery plus PDGF/IGF-1, 12 weeks postoperatively. New bone *(NB)* is present coronal to the original alveolar crest *(OB)*. New cementum *(curved arrows)* has been deposited on the root surface adjacent to the new bone. A physiologic periodontal ligament space has been regenerated. Original magnification ×40.

11-3c). Many cells were partially or completely surrounded by the new cementum. A physiologic periodontal ligament space was generated between the new cementum and new bone (Figs 11-3b and c). This space was occupied by dense connective tissue. The connective tissue fibers between the new bone and cementum were more highly organized at 5 weeks than at 2 weeks, running primarily in a vertical direction but often inserting into the new bone and cementum (Fig 11-3c). Numerous vascular channels were also present within the new periodontal ligament space. At 5 weeks minimal evidence remained of osteogenic activity within the original periodontal ligament between the old bone and tooth root in both control and treated sites. In general, the control sites exhibited

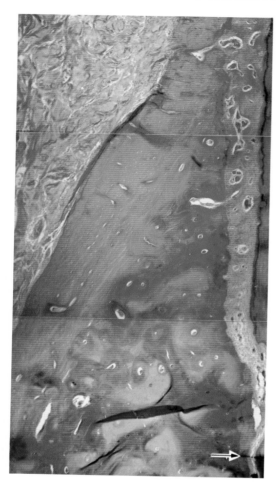

Fig 11-5a   Surgery plus PDGF/IGF-1, 24 weeks postoperatively. Dense lamellar bone is present coronal to the root notch *(arrow)*. New cementum with inserting collagen fibers is present on the root surface. A physiologic periodontal ligament is present. Original magnification ×63.

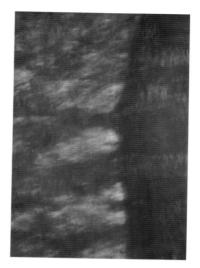

Fig 11-5b   Polarized light view of the coronal portion of the newly established periodontal ligament and tooth root. Mature collagen bundles *(white)* are oriented perpendicular to the root and insert into the root surface. Original magnification ×400.

At 12 weeks dense woven bone was present in PDGF/IGF-1–treated sites coronal to the original bone and apical extent of root planing (Fig 11-4b). The bone contained numerous osteocytes of developing haversian systems but was no longer lined by osteoblasts. New cellular cementum with inserting collagen fibers was present on the root surfaces. The periodontal ligament contained dense, well-organized collagen bundles and numerous fibroblasts and blood vessels. In control sites some new bone and cementum was present (Fig 11-4a). The density of new bone was similar to that in growth factor–treated sites but contained fewer osteocytes. The periodontal ligament in control sites also contained fewer collagen bundles and fibroblasts than the PDGF/IGF-1–treated sites. At 24 weeks, dense lamellar bone was present in all treated sites. A mature periodontal ligament was present with collagen fibers

a similar sequence of wound healing events as in treated sites, except that the time of onset was delayed, fewer osteoblastlike and cementoblastlike cells were present, and the magnitude of bone and cementum formation was significantly diminished (Fig 11-3a).

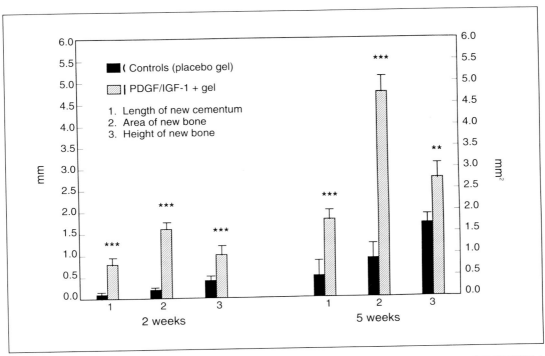

Fig 11-6    Histometric analysis of control (surgery plus placebo gel) or surgery plus gel/PDGF/IGF-1 sites. (***$P < .001$, **$P < .01$; n = 13 dogs.)

oriented perpendicular to the root surface. Sharpey's fibers could be observed in the regenerated periodontium using polarizing light (Figs 11-5a and b). The density and organization of the new bone and periodontal ligament in control sites was similar to that in the treated sites but again was less in quantity.

All specimens were coded and analyzed by standardized computer-aided histometric techniques. As shown in Fig 11-6, all three parameters measured were significantly increased ($P < .05$ to $P < .001$) in PDGF/IGF-1–treated sites compared to surgery plus placebo gel at all time points analyzed. The coronal extent of new cementum and total amount of coronal new bone were increased fivefold to tenfold by PDGF/IGF-1 treatment at 2 and 5 weeks after surgery. All parameters increased from 2 to 5 weeks.

The effects of PDGF/IGF-1 treatment on periodontal wound healing were compared to those achieved using DFDB or TCP. These studies were performed by using either DFDB (Virginia Tissue Bank) or TCP (Synthograft) into which had been mixed PDGF and IGF-1. The results of the blind histometric analysis are shown in Figs 11-7 and 11-8. At 5 weeks postoperatively, DFDB alone stimulated more new cementum and bone formation than TCP alone. Incorporation of PDGF/IGF-1 resulted in no increase in the effects of DFDB. Incorporation of PDGF/IGF-1 into TCP resulted in a two- to threefold increase in the length of new cementum and height and area of coronal new bone compared to TCP alone

193

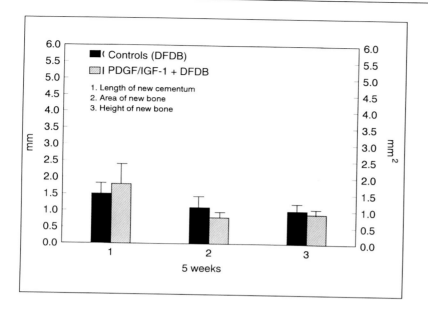

Fig 11-7    Histometric analysis of control (surgery plus demineralized freeze-dried bone [DFDB]) or surgery plus sites treated with DFDB/PDGF/IGF-1 sites (n = six dogs).

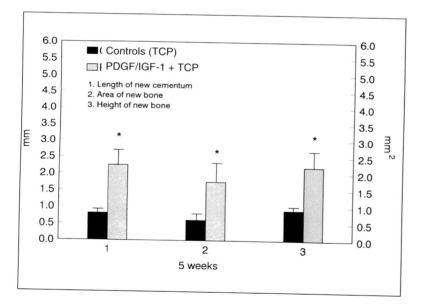

Fig 11-8    Histometric analysis of control (surgery plus beta tricalcium phosphate [TCP]) or surgery plus TCP/PDGF/IGF-1 sites (*$P < .05$; n = six dogs).

($P < .05$). When the results of these studies are compared to those obtained with use of the gel formulation, it can be seen that the combination of gel plus growth factors was more effective than were the grafting materials, either alone or pretreated with PDGF/IGF-1. Studies conducted in ligature-induced periodontal defects in cynamologous primates also have demonstrated that the PDGF/IGF-1 combination significantly enhances periodontal regeneration. Figures 11-9 a and b depict the comparisons of the results of the histometric analysis from the dog and primate studies. As

Fig 11-9a Comparison of results from control (surgery plus placebo gel) and experimental (surgery plus PDGF/IGF-1 in gel) sites in dogs with natural periodontitis and monkeys with ligature-induced attachment loss (from Giannobile et al 1994; n = 13 dogs and 10 primates).

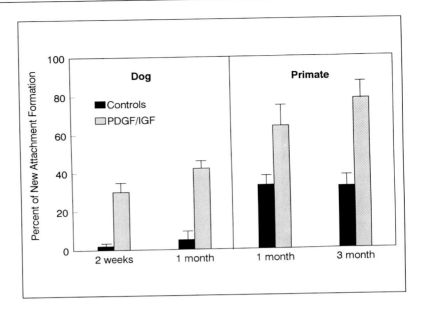

Fig 11-9b Comparison of results reported by Lynch and coworkers (1991a) using dogs with natural periodontal disease to those reported by Rutherford and coworkers (1992) using monkeys with ligature-induced attachment loss and super-infected with *P. gingivalis*. As can be seen there was a high degree of correlation in the results of the two studies.

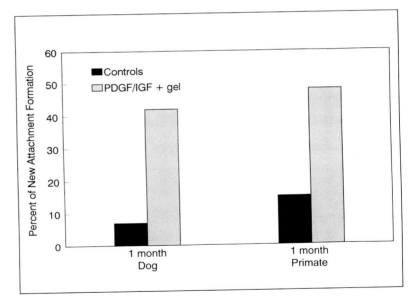

can be seen in Fig 11-9a at 3 months following surgery, sites treated with surgery plus PDGF/IGF-1 exhibited approximately 78% of the original defect healed with new attachment compared to approximately 30% new attachment in sites that received surgery plus placebo gel ($P < .01$; Giannobile et al 1994b). Rutherford and coworkers (1992) have also evaluated the effects of a gel containing PDGF/IGF-1 in nonhuman primates. The results of these studies are compared to the results reported by Lynch and coworkers in dogs with natural disease in Fig 11-9b. As can be seen there was a high degree of correlation between the results of the two studies.

## Summary

Based on the known biologic actions of growth factors, we have postulated that the combination of PDGF and IGF-1 would be effective in promoting growth of all the components of the periodontium. Extensive animal studies have indeed shown that the combination of PDGF and IGF-1 stimulates rapid osteogenesis and cementogenesis. In addition, the formation of a new functional periodontal ligament results from PDGF/IGF-1 treatment. These effects are mediated through the establishment of an increased number of osteoblasts and cementoblasts in the connective tissue region coronal to the residual alveolar crest. The number of fibroblasts from the periodontal ligament may also have been increased in the supracrestal area, but this could not be determined from these studies. When compared to current bone grafting materials used clinically (ie, DFDB and TCP), the PDGF/IGF-1 in a simple aqueous gel was more effective in increasing new cementum and alveolar bone without increasing ankylosis. By 5 weeks postoperatively there was 40.6% fill* of the periodontal defects in dogs with naturally occurring horizontal bone loss, compared to 6.9% fill* in control (surgery plus placebo gel) sites (Lynch et al 1991).

---

*Defect fill was determined by dividing the length of the complete new attachment apparatus by the length of the bone defect (cementoenamel junction to coronal extent of supporting alveolar bone) and multiplying this value by 100. Complete new attachment is defined as the coronal establishment of new cementum and alveolar bone with an interposed physiologic periodontal ligament space. Areas of new cementum without new bone or vice versa and areas of ankylosis were not included in this measurement.

## Future directions

Clearly, additional studies are necessary to evaluate the effects of the other most promising growth factors on periodontal regeneration. Even for the PDGF/IGF-1 combination, the optimum dose and optimum number of doses must still be determined. An alternative to repeated applications would be the incorporation of the growth factors into a controlled-release delivery system. Such a system might be designed to also take advantage of the principles of guided tissue regeneration. As discussed at the outset of this chapter, barrier membranes exclude nondesirable cells from the periodontal wound but do not per se stimulate desirable cells. The effects of using growth factors underneath barrier membranes deserve further study. The effects of bone growth factors on bone ingrowth around titanium implants also appear to be a fruitful area of investigation. In fact, data from a pilot study using titanium implants coated with PDGF/IGF-1 suggest that PDGF/IGF-1 can increase bone growth around dental implants (Lynch et al 1991). Additionally, the use of PDGF/IGF-1 under PTFE membranes has been shown to enhance bone growth around implants placed into fresh extraction sockets with buccal dehiscents (Becker et al 1992).

The mechanisms by which PDGF/IGF-1 (and perhaps other growth factors) act to enhance periodontal regeneration remain to be proven in vivo. Tritiated thymidine and proline labeling studies would yield valuable information on the in vivo effects of these growth factors on the proliferation, migration, and matrix synthesis of cells from the bone and periodontal ligament. The nature of the cells within the periodontal ligament that form cementum has yet to be determined. Given the rapid formation of cementum and the large number of cells on its surface following PDGF/IGF-1 treatment, the origin and nature of cementum-forming cells may be more easily studied in a model using growth factor therapy.

## Acknowledgments

The author wishes to thank Drs Ray C. Williams, Harry N. Antoniades, Gustavo Ruiz de Castilla, and Rafael Hernandez for their guidance and participation in the experimental studies described here. The experimental studies evaluating the effects of PDGF/IGF-1 on periodontal regeneration presented in this chapter were funded by NIH grant DE08878-01 and the Institute of Molecular Biology, Inc.

## References

Antoniades HN, Galanopoulos T, Neville-Golden J, Kiritsy CP, Lynch SE. Injury induces in vivo expression of platelet-derived growth factor (PDGF) and PDGF receptor in RNA's in skin epithelial cells and PDGF mRNA in connective tissue fibroblasts. Proc Natl Acad Sci USA 1991;88:565–569.

Antosz ME, Bellows CG, Aubin, JE. Effects of TGF-β and EGF on cell proliferation and formation of bone nodules in isolated fetal rat calvaria cells. J Cell Physiol 1989;140:386–395.

Assoian RK, Grotendorst GR, Muller DM, Sporn MB. Cellular transformation by coordinated action of three peptide growth factors from human platelets. Nature 1984;309:804–806.

Aukhil I, Iglhaut J. Periodontal ligament cell kinetics following experimental regenerative procedures. J Clin Periodontol 1988;15:374–82.

Becker W, Lynch SE, Lekholm U, Becker B, Caffesse R, Donath C, Sanchez R. A comparison of PTFE membranes alone or in combination with platelet-derived growth factor and insulin-like growth factor-I, or demineralized freeze-dried bone in promoting bone formation around immediate extraction socket implants: A study in dogs. J Periodontol 1993;63:929–940.

Buckley A, Davidson JM, Kamerath CD, Wolt TB, Woodward SC. Sustained release of epidermal growth factor accelerates wound repair. Proc Natl Acad Sci USA 1985;82:7340–7344.

Buser D, Hernandez R, Weber HP, Williams RC, Stich H, Lynch SE. Effect of growth factors on bone regeneration around titanium implants. J Dent Res 1991;70:301.

Canalis E, McCarthy TL, Centrella M. Growth factors and the skeletal system. J Endocrinol Invest 1989a; 12:577–584.

Canalis E, McCarthy TL, Centrella M. Effects of platelet derived growth factor on bone formation in vitro. J Cell Physiol 1989b: 140:530.

Chenu C, Pfeilschifter J, Mundy GR, Roodman GD. Transforming growth factor β inhibits formation of osteoclast-like cells in long-term human marrow cultures. Proc Natl Acad Sci USA 1988;85:5683–5687.

Cochran D, Rouse CA, Lynch SE, Graves DT. Effects of PDGF isoforms on calcium release from neonatal mouse calvaria. Bone 1993;14:53–58.

Donaldson DJ, Mahan JT. Epidermal cell migration on laminin-coated substrates. Comparison with other extracellular matrix and non-matrix proteins. Cell Tissue Res 1984;235:221–224.

Giannobile WV, Finkelman RD, Lynch SE. Comparison of canine and nonhuman primate animal models for periodontal regenerative therapy: Results following a single application of PDGF/IGF-I. J Periodontol 1994b(in press).

Gilardetti RS, Chaibi MS, Stroumza J, et al. High affinity binding of PDGF-AA and PDGF-BB to normal human osteoblasts and medulation by interleukin. Am J Physiol 1991;261(cell physiol):980–985.

Gospodarowicz D, Ferrara N, Schweigerer L, Neufeld G. Structural characterization and biological functions of fibroblast growth factor. Endocr Rev 1987; 8:95–114.

Greenhalgh DG, Sprugel KH, Murray MJ, Ross R. PDGF and FGF stimulate wound healing in the genetically diabetic mouse. Am J Pathol 1990; 136:1235–1246.

Joyce ME, Jingushi S, Scully SP, Bolander ME. Role of growth factors in fracture healing. In: Barbul A, et al, eds. Clinical and Experimental Approaches to Dermal and Epidermal Repair. New York, NY: Wiley-Liss, Inc; 1990a:391–416.

Joyce ME, Roberts AB, Sporn MB, Bolander ME. Transforming growth factor-B and the initiation of chondrogenesis and osteogenesis in the rat femur. J Cell Biol 1990b;110:2195–2207.

Kiritsy CP, Lynch SE. The role of growth factors in cutaneous wound healing: A review. Crit Rev Oral Biology Med 1993;5:21–52.

Lynch SE, Williams RC, Polson AM, et al. A combination of platelet derived and insulin-like growth factors enhances periodontal regeneration. J Clin Periodontol 1989a;16:545–548.

Lynch SE, Colvin RB, Antoniades HN. Growth factors in wound healing: single and synergistic effects on partial thickness porcine skin wounds. J Clin Invest 1989b;84:640–646.

Lynch SE. Interactions of growth factors in tissue repair. In: Barbul A, et al, eds. Clinical and Experimental Approaches to Dermal and Epidermal Repair. New York: Wiley-Liss, Inc; 1990:341–357.

Lynch SE, Williams RC. A possible role for polypeptide growth factors and differentiation factors in periodontal regeneration. Am Acad Periodontol 1990:1–5.

Lynch SE, Ruiz de Castilla G, Williams RC, et al. The effects of short term application of a combination of platelet derived and insulin-like growth factors on periodontal wound healing. J Periodontol 1991;62:458–467.

Lynch SE, Buser D, Hernandez RA, et al. Effects of platelet-derived growth factory insulin-like growth factor -I combination on bone regeneration around titanium dental implants. *J Periodontol* 1991;88: 565–569.

Lynch SE, Giannobile WV, Polypeptide growth factors: Molecular mediators of tissue repair. In Genco RJ (ed). Molecular Pathogenesis of Periodontal Diseases. Washington DC: ASM Publications (in press).

Matsuda N, Lin W-L, Kumar MI, Genco RJ. Mitogenic, chemotactic and synthetic responses of rat periodontal ligament cells to polypeptide growth factors in vitro. *J Periodontol* 1992;63:515–525.

Pfeilschifter J, Oechsner M, Naumann A, Gronwald RGK, Minne HW, Ziegler R. Stimulation of bone matrix apposition in vitro by local growth factors: a comparison between insulin-like growth factor I, platelet-derived growth factor, and transforming growth factor β. *Endocrinology* 1990;127:69–75.

Pfeilschifter J, Wolf O, Naumann A, et al. Chemotactic response of osteoblastlike cells to transforming growth factor beta. *J Bone Miner Res* 1990;5:825–830.

Piché JE, Graves DT. Study of the growth factor requirements of human bone-derived cells: a comparison with human fibroblasts. *Bone* 1989;10: 131–138.

Pierce GF. Tissue repair and growth factors. In: *Encyclopedia of Human Biology* 7:1991 (in press).

Rutherford AB, Niekresh CR, Kennedy JE, Charette MF. Platelet-derived and insulin-like growth factors stimulate regeneration of periodontal attachment in monkeys. *J Periodont Res* 1992;27: 285–290.

Schultz GS, White M, Mitchell R, et al. Epithelial wound healing enhanced by transforming growth factor alpha and vaccinia growth factor. *Science* 1987;235:350–352.

Selvig KA, Wikesjö UME, Bogle GC, Finkelman RD. Impaired early bone formation in periodontal fenestration defects in dogs following application of insulin-like growth factor II, basic fibroblast growth factor and transforming growth factor B. *J Clin Periodont* 1994 (in press).

Tashjian AH, Voelkel EF, Lazzaro M, et al. Alpha and beta human transforming growth factors stimulate prostaglandin production and bone resorption in cultured mouse calvaria. *Proc Natl Acad Sci USA* 1985;82:4543–4548.

Terranova VP, Hic S, Franzetti L, Lyall RM, Wikesjö UME. A biological approach to periodontal regeneration — AFSCM: assays for specific cell migration. *J Periodontol* 1987;58:247–257.

Woodley D, Bachmann PM, O'Keefe EJ. The role of matrix components in human keratinocyte re-epithelialization. In Barbul A, et al, eds. *Clinical and Experimental Approaches to Dermal and Epidermal Repair.* New York: Wiley-Liss, Inc; 1990:129–140.

# Chapter 12

# Augmentation of Periodontal Regeneration Response Using Biologic Mediators

Giovanpaolo Pini Prato / Carlo Clauser / Pierpaolo Cortellini

A fibrin-fibronectin sealing system (FFSS) has been commercially available (Tissucol-Tisseel, Immuno AG, Vienna, Austria) in Europe since 1975. It was developed to improve the results of microsurgery on peripheral nerves by providing hemostasis, gluing of the severed neural fibers, and enhancement of the biologic response in the early phases of wound healing (Matras and Kuderna 1975). This FFSS preparation has since been used in several fields of surgery (Schlag and Redl 1986). It is a human plasma cryoprecipitate, which consists of highly concentrated fibrinogen, fibronectin, factor XIII, platelet-derived growth factor (PDGF), and antiplasmins. Small amounts of plasminogen are also present. Aprotinin (a bovine antiplasmin), thrombin, and calcium chloride are added at the moment of use. Activated thrombin induces the clotting of the cryoprecipitate. Aprotinin in different concentrations can modulate the stability of the artificial clot. In any case, the clot is locally degraded and completely absorbed (Pini Prato et al 1985; Seelich 1982).

Highly concentrated fibrinogen, fibronectin, and PDGF play a significant role not only in the coagulation process, but also in wound healing.

## Biologic mediators in periodontal surgery

A series of experimental and clinical trials in periodontal surgery have been undertaken in the past decade. They were based on positive results achieved in several fields of surgery and on the knowledge of the activities of these biologic mediators, which will be discussed later in some detail. The investigations can be divided into three main groups, whose character and aims varied according to the evolution of the general knowledge about wound healing in periodontal literature. In the first group, the focus was not on regeneration but on the adhesive effect, the hemostasis, and the quality and speed of wound healing. In the second group, the focus was on new connective tissue attachment. In the third group, the information gathered from the preceding studies was used to investigate the effects of these biologic mediators on the tissue response to guided tissue regeneration procedures.

## Use of FFSS in conventional periodontal surgery

A preliminary clinical investigation assessed the feasibility of using this fibrin-fibronectin sealing system in human periodontal surgery (Bartolucci and Pini Prato 1982). The technique used for applying the FFSS was shown in a free gingival graft and a lateral pedicle flap. Further studies were aimed at assessing the expected advantages of the same FFSS used in several surgical procedures. Gluing the flaps seemed to be remarkably easier and quicker than suturing them. The clinical results obtained from apically positioned flaps, modified Widman flaps, free gingival grafts, and sliding flaps were evaluated in surgically treated patients. No adverse effects were observed 3 to 12 months after surgery. It was concluded that all surgical procedures had been facilitated without any apparent adverse effect (Pini Prato et al 1983, 1986).

An experimental study was carried out on dogs (Pini Prato et al 1985) using the FFSS to close periodontal flaps. Histologic examination revealed a denser and more homogeneous coagulum the day after surgery on the test (ie, FFSS) side. Higher concentration and better organization of fibroblasts in periodontal wounds were found at 3 and 7 days postoperatively, compared to the contralateral control sites, which had undergone the same procedure but without the fibrin-fibronectin sealing system.

The results of this experiment were confirmed on the replantation model by Nasjleti et al (1986), who used a lyophilized autologous plasma (LAP) in rhesus monkeys. Lyophilized autologous protein contains fibronectin, fibrinogen, and factor XIIIa; the qualitative composition closely resembles that of the FFSS used in the earlier experiment. In the first 45 days after surgery, it was observed that LAP "enhances healing by early replacement of the fibrin clot, increased connective tissue cell proliferation, reduction of the inflammatory response and inhibition of root cementum resorption."

A split-mouth clinical study was carried out on 51 patients over 3 years to compare the results after different types of periodontal wounds were closed with silk sutures or FFSS (Pini Prato et al 1987). The FFSS was easier and quicker to use than sutures and provided better early hemostasis as well as the complete adhesion of the wound surface of the flaps or grafts to their surgical bed. On the control side, inflammation was observed around sutures. The FFSS appeared to be associated with a more rapid maturation of the healing tissues.

In these early periodontal applications of the FFSS, its mechanical and hemostatic qualities were used only to fix flaps or grafts without sutures, thereby facilitating surgery, preventing hematomas, saving chair time, and enhancing patient comfort. The biologic effects of the fibrin-fibronectin sealing system were observed in the early phases of wound healing: the fibroblasts appeared to colonize the wounds more rapidly and effectively in the connective tissue and bone of experimental animals. Clinically, the absence of inflammation around the sutures and an apparently quicker maturation of the tissues led to the conclusion that the FFSS could be especially helpful in delicate procedures where even small amounts of inflammatory infiltrate could have a significant effect on the outcome of surgery, as in tiny sliding flaps or free gingival grafts over denuded roots. In this case the mechanical adhesion to the whole recipient area could also be beneficial. Additional advantages could stem from the stability of the flap on the root surface in the most critical areas (eg, flap adapted against a root surface).

## Fibrin-fibronectin sealing system and new connective tissue attachment

*The biologic mediators.* The substances contained in the FFSS contribute to the coagulation process and also play an important role in the regeneration of connective tissue. Their effects on periodontal wound healing have been studied with special emphasis on the connective tissue attachment level. The discussion of the effects of biologic mediators in this chapter is limited to the substances contained in the FFSS, with which the authors have direct experience.

*Fibrinogen* is a high-molecular-weight (340,000 daltons) protein, which is transformed into fibrin by thrombin to form the bulk of the blood clot, thereby providing hemostasis. It is arranged to form a network, linking collagen and glycosaminoglycans in such a way that tissue adhesion occurs. Later, the fibroblasts colonize the clot and repair the wound; fibroblast adhesion and multiplication are promoted by fibrin and factor XIIIa (Caton et al 1986).

*Fibronectin* is a high-molecular-weight (450,000 daltons) glycoprotein. The most relevant knowledge about fibronectin has been reviewed by Polson and Proye (1983) and more recently by Terranova and Wikesjö (1987) and Mendieta et al (1990). Fibronectin is found in plasma, on the cell surface, in the extracellular matrix, and in the basement membrane of epithelium. It forms covalent links to different types of collagen and to fibrin, which enables fibronectin to play a role in the early phase of wound healing, forming a substrate for factor XIIIa in a clot. Fibronectin promotes cell-to-cell adhesion and cell mobility. It plays an important role in promoting and regulating cell-matrix interaction. In particular, fibronectin promotes migration, adhesion, attachment, and the synthetic activity of fibroblasts.

*Factor XIII* is a transglutaminase, an enzyme that mediates the links between fibrin and fibronectin in the clot and between the clot and the collagen and glycosaminoglycans of the connective tissue.

*Plasminogen* is a glycoprotein (90,000 daltons) that is transformed into plasmin under the effect of active thrombin. The proteasic activity of plasmin causes the lysis of fibrin and fibronectin, thereby destroying the clot. Plasminogen is closely associated with fibrinogen. The plasminogen-fibrinogen ratio in Tissucol is reduced up to 30 times less than in human plasma. This reduced proportion is more favorable to clot stability.

*Antiplasmins* are macroglobulins that modulate the rate of coagulum lysis, inhibiting plasmin activity.

*Thrombin* is a serinoprotease (40,000 dalton) that activates fibrinogen and factor XIII in the presence of $Ca^{++}$, which is provided as calcium chloride in Tissucol. Thrombin stimulates the growth of fibroblasts and the synthesis of fibronectin and collagen (Caton et al 1986). In the commercially available FFSS, aprotinin is added to further stabilize the clot. Aprotinin is a polypeptide extracted from bovine lungs, and it inhibits plasmin activity.

*Platelet-derived growth factor* (PDGF) is the major human serum polypeptide growth factor (Lynch et al 1987). Polypeptide growth factors are a class of natural biologic response modifiers that can stimulate and regulate a variety of biologic processes, such as proliferation, differentiation, mobility and matrix synthesis of the cells (Terranova and Wikesjö 1987). Platelet-derived growth factor is stored in alpha granules of circulating platelets and is released into the serum during blood clotting. It is a potent mitogen and chemoattractant for fibroblast and arterial smooth muscle cells; it also stimulates the synthesis of collagenase and of specific types of collagen by fibroblasts (Lynch et al 1987).

*Experimental evidence in periodontology.* The role of fibrin was investigated by Polson and Proye (1983) in a replantation model. A fibrin linkage preceded the formation of collagen fiber attachment to the root surface, apparently preventing epithelium from migrating apically on demineralized root surfaces. The formation of this early fibrin linkage could involve other biologic mediators. Fibronectin might serve to anchor a blood clot to collagen, being covalently linked to fibrin and collagen by factor XIIIa (activated).

The activity of fibronectin has been studied in vivo and in vitro on fibroblasts and especially on periodontal ligament cells. Studies in vitro have shown that the presence of fibronectin increases the attachment of fibroblasts to periodontally diseased, scaled, and root-planed root surfaces (Fernyhough and Page 1983; Terranova and Martin 1982).

In vivo studies were carried out by performing flap surgery on different species. Caffesse et al (1985) found that areas treated with a combination of citric acid and exogenous fibronectin showed remarkably greater connective tissue reattachment than areas treated with either agent alone or left untreated, after mucoperiosteal flap surgery in dogs. Fibronectin alone did not significantly enhance the results of surgery.

Ripamonti et al (1987) stated that the potential for connective tissue attachment and bone regeneration may be enhanced if a surgically exposed root surface — planed, notched and demineralized with citric acid — is additionally treated with specific attachment glycoproteins (ie, exogenous fibronectin) and plasma factors.

Other studies were performed using the replantation model. Caton et al (1986) tried

the FFSS (Tissucol) to evaluate its effects on periodontal wound healing in monkeys. The study was carried out on the labial surfaces of premolars and molars. All the extracted teeth were root planed. One group was replanted, a second group was treated with an application of tissue adhesive to the planed surface prior to replantation, and a third group underwent citric acid decalcification of the planed root surfaces before application of tissue adhesive and replantation. Seven days after surgery, the first and second groups showed junctional epithelium up to the reference notch, with no sign of new attachment. In contrast, the teeth that were decalcified prior to application of the tissue adhesive demonstrated fiber attachment to planed root surfaces and little or no epithelial downgrowth. It was concluded that the commercially available fibrin-fibronectin sealing system did not per se promote periodontal regeneration. On the other hand, the tissue adhesive did not affect wound healing adversely, even in the replantation model. The tissue adhesive did not enhance the new attachment after replantation but could be useful to achieve mechanical stability after flap surgery.

On the other hand, Nasjleti et al (1986) observed enhanced connective tissue attachment after treatment of lyophilized autologous plasma on scaled root surfaces, even without citric acid treatment, using the replantation monkey model. It should be stressed that the biologic mediators (FFSS and LAP) were not identical in the last two experiments; this could account for the different outcomes.

In conclusion, the results of histologic analyses on single roots indicated a positive role played by fibronectin alone, or by fibronectin plus citric acid, in producing new connective tissue attachment. In contrast, the results of experiments on furcation areas in beagle dogs yielded negative results, even in combination with citric acid treatment (Smith et al 1987; Wikesjö et al 1988).

In the aforementioned studies, the effect of fibronectin had been investigated in the healing between tissues and denuded and/or demineralized root surface, without interposed cementum. More recently, Mendieta et al (1990) also investigated the conditions that favor the sorption and retention of fibronectin to human root cementum in vitro. The results of this study indicated that fibronectin sorption to cementum was "rapid, electrostatic in nature, competitive, reversible, $Ca^{++}$ facilitated and maximized by prior treatment of the root with citric acid and sodium hypochlorite." This fact suggests that a similar mechanism could also account for the usually better results achieved by combined treatment with fibronectin and citric acid of scaled root surfaces.

The effects of fibronectin alone or in combination with other substances have also been studied, specifically on periodontal ligament cells in vitro. Terranova et al (1987) reported that fibronectin and endothelial cell growth factor (EGF) could contribute to periodontal regeneration by inducing attachment, migration, and proliferation of periodontal ligament cells.

Furthermore, fibronectin has synergistic activity in combination with other substances. For example, basic fibroblast growth factor (bFGF) proved to be a powerful chemoattractant and a mitogen for periodontal ligament cells (Terranova et al 1989). The combination of fibronectin and bFGF was a marginally more potent attractant than bFGF alone (Terranova et al 1989).

Fibrinogen, fibronectin, and plasma factor XIII affect periodontal wound healing positively. And PDGF, even if present only in small amounts in FFSS, may also influence the clinical results. It has been demonstrated that purified PDGF enhances the repair of the soft tissue wounds in vivo.

This effect was even more marked if insulinlike growth factors (IGF-1) were added (Lynch et al 1987). This association proved to enhance regeneration of periodontal structures in beagle dogs, with the formation of new cementumlike deposits and alveolar bone (Lynch et al 1989).

*Clinical studies.* The possibility of gaining new attachment by the use of biologic mediators has been tried clinically as well. Caffesse et al (1988) evaluated the effects of citric acid demineralization and autologous fibronectin application with Widman flap procedures on 29 patients, using a split-mouth design. Clinical probing attachment gain was observed on both test and control sides but was greater on the test side, where citric acid and fibronectin had been applied.

Yeung and Boyatzis (1990) investigated attachment gain after treatment of through-and-through furcation lesions. They were not able to find any significant difference between sites treated with autologous fibronectin and citric acid and sites treated with citric acid alone. This result is in agreement with the experimental results of Wikesjö et al (1988) and Smith et al (1987) on the furcation model.

## Fibrin-fibronectin sealing system and guided tissue regeneration procedures

In the late 1980s, the use of guided tissue regeneration (GTR) procedure became widespread. Subsequently the use of FFSS in conjunction with microporous filters was considered. The rationale for using this combination was based on biologic and mechanical considerations. The biologic aspects have been discussed under the heading "Fibrin-fibronectin sealing system and new connective tissue attachment." In summary, biologic mediators enhanced the connective tissue gain, at least in some instances. In any case, they did not produce unfavorable side effects. A beneficial effect could therefore be reasonably expected when FFSS is used in combination with membranes for GTR procedures. The mechanical aspects could be even more significant for clinical results.

Several mechanical problems may be significant for regeneration: the stability of the clot, the stability of the flap and of the membrane, and the need for space for the regenerating tissues. Egelberg (1987) expressed the need to develop surgical techniques that would provide improved protection of the healing wound and enhanced adhesion and maturation of the coagulum at the root surface, as well as repopulation of root surface by cells originating from the periodontal ligament. If the risk of mechanical rupture and contamination at the root surface–coagulum interface is kept under control, the oral epithelium is not likely to gain early access to this interface. The FFSS provides an artificial clot that is very stable 3 minutes after application and persists longer than the natural coagulum because of the presence of anti-fibrinolytic substances.

The need for stability in surgical flaps was emphasized by Caton et al (1986). The fibrin linkage to demineralized root surfaces is well protected in the replantation model, whereas it could be disrupted in clinical applications because of poor flap adaptation and/or flap movement. The tissue-adhesive protein did not enhance attachment gain in the replantation model but could be helpful in strengthening and protecting the fibrin linkage in periodontal flap surgery. The FFSS provides immediate stability by means of an artificial clot. This is not a synthetic glue, but it has the same qualitative composition as the natural clot and shares its elastic behavior. The resulting homogeneous environment prevents the separation of the flap and the recipient area, even in cases of mild mechanical injuries, whereas cyanoacrylates or other synthetic gluing materials

cause separation of tissues even after slight muscle contraction.

Another factor considered significant for successful regeneration is the stability of the membranes in guided tissue regeneration procedures; in fact, the stability of the membrane has been a concern since the beginning of this type of surgery and in the first reported case (Nyman et al 1982) a resin was used to fix the membrane to the tooth. Since then, various materials and techniques have been used (Becker et al 1987; Gottlow et al 1986). The FFSS provides an additional immediate and persistent means of fixing the membrane; it helps in determining the exact position of the membrane, but it is advisable to use it in combination with sutures to prevent movement in case of injury.

A more subtle mechanical issue has been clearly pointed out by Gottlow et al (1986), who stated that no bone regeneration can be achieved if no space is left for the regenerating bone, despite the formation of new cementum and new connective fibers inserted in it. This space can be lacking because of a too-close positioning of the membrane relative to the root surface, or it can decrease during the healing process because of postoperative recession (Gottlow et al 1986). A fibrin-fibronectin clot can be inserted to fill a defect, maintaining a predetermined amount of space for regeneration while supporting and stabilizing the membrane and the flap.

In conclusion, the FFSS fills the defect, maintains the space for regeneration, and stabilizes the membrane (Fig 12-1). Furthermore, it helps to stabilize the surgical flap that covers the healing would.

## Clinical results on angular bone defects and furcation involvements

Because biologic mediators were reported to effectively obtain attachment gain, and

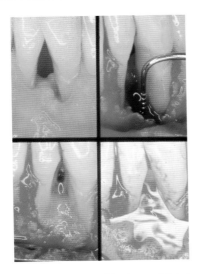

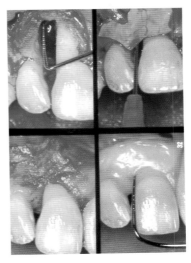

Fig 12-1 The defect is filled with the artificial clot, which supports the membrane, thereby maintaining the necessary space for the regenerating tissues.

Fig 12-2 *Top:* Angular bone defect treated by a Millipore filter and a fibrin-fibronectin sealing system. *Bottom:* Reentry after 3 months and final healing after free gingival graft.

because the available FFSS fulfilled the mechanical requirements for optimal healing, there seemed to be a sufficient theoretical basis to try the FFSS in combination with membranes for GTR. This therapeutic association has been used in some challenging situations.

Fibrin-fibronectin sealing system was first used to treat a severe iatrogenic defect (Pini Prato et al 1988). A combination one-, two-, and three-walled osseous defect was evident extending almost to the apex of a maxillary right central incisor distally. The 14-mm pocket was associated with a chronic abscess caused by an orthodontic elastic band, which had been lost in the sulcus 6 years earlier. After combined treatment by means of a Millipore filter and fibrin-fibronectin sealing system, an 11-mm bone fill of the defect was measured at the reentry procedure after 3 months (Figs 12-2 and 12-3). The filling of the infrabony defect was quite satisfactory and was associated with a regrowth of crestal bone up to

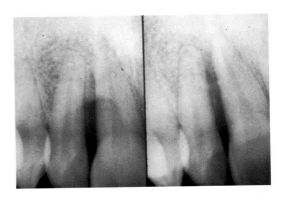

Fig 12-3 Same patient as in Fig 12-2: radiographic examination. *Left:* Preoperative view. *Right:* Bone regeneration after 6 months.

3 mm (distobuccal angle) and slight resorption (1 mm) only at the mesiobuccal angle and in the interproximal space. The mobility was degree 2 before treatment and became degree 0 at the reentry. The iatrogenic etiology and the age of the patient could have favored the positive outcome of

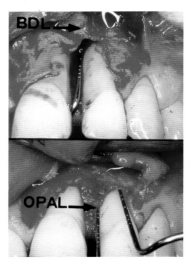

Fig 12-4 *Top:* Angular bone defect. The arrow indicates the most apical extension of the defect *(BDL). Bottom:* Open probing at the same site 8 weeks after guided tissue regeneration procedure. The arrow indicates the most apical extension of the residual defect *(OPAL).*

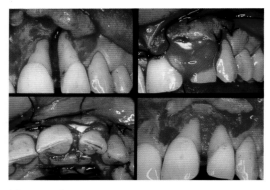

Fig 12-5 Same patient as in Fig 12-4. The artificial clot that fills the defect supports and stabilizes the membrane. Healing after 8 weeks.

Table 12-1    Average % open probing attachment gain (OPAG) in guided tissue regeneration (GTR) plus fibrin-fibronectin sealing system (FFSS) sites versus GTR alone sites*

| Infrabony defects | GTR + FFSS sites | | GTR sites | |
|---|---|---|---|---|
| | n | % OPAG | n | % OPAG |
| Two-walled | 1 | 68.67 | 4 | 41.31 |
| Three-walled | 1 | 61.25 | 21 | 50.91 |
| One-, two-, and three-walled | 3 | 52.31 | 5 | 48.31 |
| Total (mean) | 5 | (57.37) | 30 | (49.20) |

*Two one-walled defects were treated by GTR alone, while no one-walled defect was treated by GTR + FFSS. Therefore only 35 of 37 bone defects are reported in this table.

this treatment. The use of FFSS was helpful in facilitating the positioning and stabilization of the membranes and of the flaps. Certainly it did not hamper the result. However, some problems remained unsolved after the GTR procedure. The preoperative recession had slightly worsened and required further treatment, namely a free gingival graft for root coverage. Gingival recession during healing is an acknowledged problem of GTR procedures (Gottlow et al 1986).

Cortellini et al (1990) reported the results observed in 39 patients, in whom 68 periodontal defects were treated by guided tissue regeneration procedures using different porous materials. The bone lesions were classified as angular bone defects (n = 37), bone craters (n = 4), bone dehiscences (n = 6), and furcation involvements (n = 21). The furcation lesions were classified either as second degree (n = 6) or third degree (n = 15).

To evaluate the results of the procedures, clinical qualitative judgments and probe measurements were used. The following measurements were recorded: *(1)* during the first surgical procedure and after

Table 12-2 Filling of infrabony defects treated with guided tissue regeneration (GTR) + fibrin-fibronectin sealing system (FFSS) and with guided tissue regeneration (GTR) alone (same patients as in Table 12-1)

| Infrabony defects | GTR + FFSS sites | | | | GTR sites | | | |
|---|---|---|---|---|---|---|---|---|
| | | Amount of fill* | | | | Amount of fill | | |
| | n | C | P | F | n | C | P | F |
| Two-walled | 1 | 1 | 0 | 0 | 4 | 2 | 2 | 0 |
| Three-walled | 1 | 1 | 0 | 0 | 21 | 19 | 2 | 0 |
| One-, two-, three-walled | 3 | 2 | 1 | 0 | 5 | 2 | 3 | 0 |
| Total | 5 | 4 | 1 | 0 | 30 | 23 | 7 | 0 |

*C = complete; P = partial (at least 50%); F = failure (<50% of the initial defect).

thorough debridement, the most apical extension of the bone defect, from the cementoenamel junction or restoration (BDL); and (2) during the reentry procedure, the measurements were taken at the same sites as in (1), whereby the open probing attachment level (OPAL) was recorded (Fig 12-4). Using the above data, the open probing attachment gain (OPAG) was computed by subtracting the OPAL from the BDL at each site. Finally, the percentage of the original defect covered by the postoperative open probing new attachment (percent OPAG) was computed using the following formula:

$$\% \text{ OPAG} = (\text{OPAG} \times 100)/\text{BDL}$$

These measurements were taken to gain information about the biologic effects of different procedures and materials. The clinical evaluation (complete filling, partial filling, failure) was aimed at obtaining information on the predictability of clinical success of these procedures.

Five of 37 angular bone defects were treated with the use of a fibrin-fibronectin sealing system (Fig 12-5). The percent OPAG values obtained with and without the fibrin-fibronectin sealing system in each type of angular bone defect are compared in Table 12-1. A similar comparison

was made between the clinical evaluations of the two groups (Table 12-2). In evaluating the data for guided tissue regeneration with and without FFSS in this case series, it should be noted that a comparison of the two methods was not the aim of the study. The original purpose of the authors was to show how little the results of GTR procedures appeared to vary when different types of membranes were used. The analysis reported here was performed based on the original data after publication of the study.

The percent OPAG is consistently higher in the GTR group in which the fibrin-fibronectin sealing system was used than in the GTR group without FFSS (Table 12-1). The comparison of the clinical evaluations follows the same trend (Table 12-2). These results suggest a beneficial role of fibronectin, fibrin, and PDGF in enhancing connective tissue regeneration. The data are not sufficient to support this hypothesis, however, because the small size of the sample and the nonrandom assignment of the treatments preclude a sound statistical inference. However, the bias is against FFSS, because this was used in the most difficult cases, especially when special mechanical problems were encountered. The results were equal or better when FFSS was used, despite this

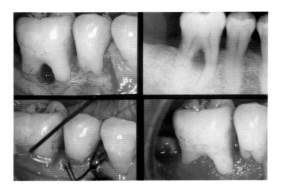

Fig 12-6 Class III furcation involvement treated by fibrin-fibronectin sealing system and two polytetrafluoroethylene membranes. Healing at 6 weeks.

bias in the assignment of cases. This observation would again support the hypothesis of a beneficial role of FFSS. This hypothesis is also in agreement with the data of Nasjleti et al (1986), which indicated more enhanced healing in sites treated with LAP than in control sites, after replantation. If fibronectin, fibrin, and factor XIII enhance attachment gain in flap procedures, they could also be beneficial in GTR procedures. Experimental research on standardized defects is needed to assess whether there is a real advantage when FFSS is used in combination with GTR procedures and if this advantage is based on its mechanical or biologic properties.

The results of GTR procedures on class III furcation involvements were considered unpredictable. Pontoriero et al (1987) reported complete closure of class III furcations in four of 16 treated cases, partial healing in nine, and failure in three cases. In the authors' experience, the clinical results after single surgical treatment fell in equal proportions: complete filling (5), partial filling (5), and failure (5) (Cortellini et al 1990). The only furcation treated with GTR plus FFSS in this series was a class III mandibular molar furcation, and this result-

ed in complete fill (Fig 12-6). Three other cases of class III furcations were treated thereafter by the authors with GTR plus FFSS: two were partial fillings and one was complete filling at the time of membrane removal. Again, these cases suggest a beneficial role of FFSS in the treatment of class III furcations by means of GTR procedures, but this conclusion is based on only four cases. Moreover, the treatment of through-and-through furcations by demineralization and fibronectin application, without GTR, did not result in enhanced attachment gain in dogs (Smith et al 1987; Wikesjö et al 1988) or in humans (Yeung and Boyatzis 1990).

A study was carried out (Cortellini et al 1991) to compare the results of GTR procedures with and without the use of FFSS in the treatment of infrabony defects in humans. Thirteen pairs of controlateral teeth with similar one-, two-, and three-wall combination defects were selected in 13 patients for intraindividual comparison. Each defect in each patient was randomly assigned to one of the two treatment groups (Figs 12-7 and 12-8). Baseline measurements (before surgery) included probing attachment level (PAL) and probing pocket depth (PPD). Intrasurgical measurements included the distance between cementoenamel junction (CEJ) and the bottom of the defect (CEJ-BD) and the distance between CEJ and the interproximal bone crest (CEJ-BC). The infrabony component of the defects was computed by subtracting CEJ-BC from CEJ-BD. On both the test and control sides an ePTFE membrane (GORE periodontal material, WL Gore & Associates, Flagstaff, AZ) was positioned after root planing and defect debridement. On the test side only, FFSS was used to fill the defect under the membrane. The membranes were removed 4 to 6 weeks postoperatively. Probing attachment level and probing pocket depth were measured again 1 year postoperatively,

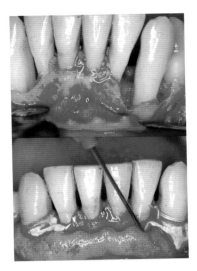 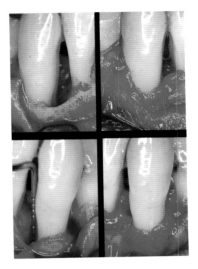

Fig 12-7  *Top:* Symmetric angular bone defects on the mesial aspects of the mandibular canines. *Bottom:* Membranes cover both defects, while the fibrin-fibronectin sealing system is used only on the left side (test side).

Fig 12-8  Same patient as in Fig 12-7. *Top:* The right canine before and after the GTR procedure. *Bottom:* The left canine before and after the same treatment, with the addtion of fibrin-fibronectin sealing system.

Table 12-3  Descriptive statistics (mean ± SD) of the changes in clinical and intrasurgical measurements between baseline and 1-year visits

| Side | PAL gain | PPD reduction | Bone gain |
|------|----------|---------------|-----------|
| Test side | 4.4 ± 2.0 | 6.9 ± 2.9 | 4.6 ± 1.8 |
| Control side | 3.3 ± 1.1 | 5.1 ± 2.3 | 3.5 ± 1.5 |

immediately before a reentry procedure. A full-thickness flap was raised to expose bone, and CEJ-BD and CEJ-BC were measured again. The results are summarized in Table 12-3. Both treatments yielded positive results in terms of PAL gain, bone gain, and PPD reduction, confirming the effectiveness of GTR treatment in angular bony defects (Cortellini et al 1993a). The average improvement of the periodontal parameters was greater on the test (FFSS) side, but the difference did not reach the threshold of statistical significance in this limited sample.

This study confirmed the results obtained by Caffesse et al (1991) on dogs. The results of both studies suggest that FFSS may play a positive role, but the associated improvement in healing was not remarkable, because it did not produce significant differences in the reported human and animal studies, in which the sample sizes were small.

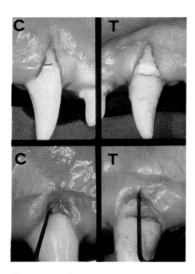

Fig 12-9 Symmetric surgically induced recessions in dogs. *Top*: Control *(C)* and test *(T)* sides after surgery. *Bottom*: The same recessions after 4 months of plaque accumulation.

## Treatment of buccal recessions

Because the association of GTR and FFSS appeared to work well in angular bone defects, it was tempting to try it in the most critical situation, namely gingival recession. On the other hand, no data were available to warrant the application of the GTR principle (without FFSS) to the treatment of buccal recession, even if its effectiveness was well documented for cases of angular bony defects and class II furcations (Caffesse et al 1990; Gottlow et al 1986; Pontoriero et al 1988). Moreover, there was the risk that the membrane would induce damage to the soft tissue during healing, especially if the tissue was thin.

Gottlow et al (1986) stated that the root surface area, which is available for periodontal ligament cell repopulation, can

decrease depending on "the degree of gingival recession that occurs during healing": this implies that a certain amount of gingival recession does occur in the postoperative period after GTR procedures. In fact, in a series of 68 patients, three patients showed remarkable postoperative gingival recession (Cortellini et al 1990). One patient required free gingival graft for root coverage. In another patient, an ulcer was evident over the coronal border of the Millipore membrane during the healing phase. Thus, the literature and our previous experience suggested that membranes could induce, rather than treat, recessions.

A critical factor in the successful treatment of recession could be identified in the difficulty of providing the necessary space for the regenerating tissues in an unfavorable nutritional environment, ie, a root surface in front of a membrane without direct blood supply. Another problem can arise from mechanical interference of the membrane border with a thin covering flap, which is already in critical condition because its nutritional supply is reduced by the presence of the membrane itself. In this situation, a fibrin-fibronectin sealing system could be useful because of its biologic activity and even more so because of its mechanical properties, because it maintains room for regeneration and prevents movement of the membrane against the flap.

Based on these considerations, an experiment was carried out to assess the possibility of obtaining new connective tissue attachment to correct buccal recessions by means of a GTR procedure (Cortellini et al 1991). The outline of the experiment was as follows. Soft tissue and bone were dissected to create a recession on the buccal aspect of maxillary canines in three dogs, using preformed templates to obtain lesions of the same size and shape on both sides of each animal. A coronal notch was made at the cementoenamel junction. Plaque was

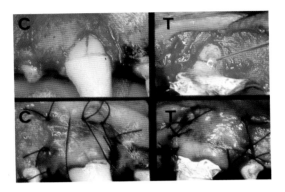

Fig 12-10 Treatment of the experimental recessions shown in Fig 12-9. *Top:* Application of the fibrin-fibronectin sealing system (both sides) and of a polytetrafluoroethylene membrane on the test *(T)* side only. *Bottom:* Sliding flaps cover both recessions.

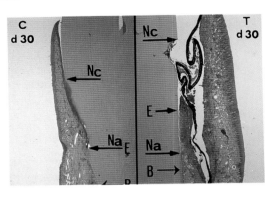

Fig 12-11 Histologic sections 30 days postoperatively. *(left)* Long junctional epithelium on the control *(C)* side. *(right)* Significant new connective tissue attachment *(Nc)* over the reference apical notch *(Na)* on the test *(T)* side. *E* = most apical epithelial cells; *B* = bone crest.

allowed to accumulate for 4 months (Fig 12-9). After this period, the recessions were carefully scaled and planed to eliminate debris and cementum. Then daily oral hygiene was administered for 1 month. Finally, all the defects were treated surgically. A pedicle flap was dissected and reflected exposing the bone crest. A sulcus was made to mark the bone crest level on the root. This V-shaped sulcus formed a triangular area with the cementoenamel junction sulcus. On the test side, a polytetrafluoroethylene membrane was positioned to cover the recession, the FFSS was injected between the membrane and the root surface, and the pedicle flap was sutured at the cementoenamel junction to cover the recession. On the contralateral control side, the same procedure was performed, except for the membrane application (Fig 12-10). The animals were killed at 15, 30, or 50 days. At histometric evaluation, the areas covered by new connective tissue were strikingly larger on the test side where the GTR procedure with FFSS had been used (Fig 12-11). The percentage of the original recession (between the reference notches) that was

covered by new connective tissue attachment on the test side ranged from 23.23% to 39.36%, while on the control side the values ranged from 0.46% to 6.15%, showing that a GTR procedure associated with biologic mediators is effective in achieving new connective tissue attachment in an experimental buccal recession. Even so, the result was far from a complete success: only about one quarter to one third of the original recession was lined with new connective tissue attachment.

The aim of the above-described experiment was to assess whether it was possible to treat buccal recessions by means of a GTR procedure, although clinical experience and literature seemed to indicate the contrary. To meet this goal, FFSS was used in combination with membranes on the test side. The control side was treated by FFSS without a membrane to exclude the possibility that biologic mediators and not the membrane was responsible for regeneration. The FFSS alone did not achieve the result, but it may have contributed to the positive result on the test side (FFSS plus GTR), at least by keeping the membrane separate from the prominent root surface. At the time of the experiment, the treatment by membrane alone appeared to be doomed to failure and was not taken into consideration even as a control. This experiment demonstrated that new connective tissue attachment can be achieved also on buccal recession by a GTR procedure associated with the use of a FFSS. This combination maintains room for regeneration, may help in protecting the covering flap, and could also enhance the early phase of healing. The clinical implication of the encouraging experimental result was clear: the association of FFSS and membranes was promising in the treatment of buccal recession.

During the same period, evidence was published (Tinti and Vincenzi 1990) of favorable clinical results in the treatment of buccal recession by GTR procedures without using biologic mediators. The authors used a semilunar bipedicled flap coronally positioned on the membrane to cover the recession. The flap could consist either of keratinized tissue or alveolar mucosa. A polytetrafluoroethylene membrane was interposed between the flap and the root. The membrane was applied and sutured in such a way that it could not collapse onto the root surfaces, thereby obtaining space for the regenerating tissues. The clinical results were excellent, with complete root coverage. Based on the general theory of GTR and on the results of our experiment on buccal recessions, one could expect that these cases resulted in truly new connective tissue attachment. These clinical results also provide a suitable explanation for the experimental evidence on dogs' recessions. In fact, it is not clear whether the mechanical aspects alone are responsible for the observed success of GTR in association with biologic mediators. This hypothesis would be supported by the excellent clinical results obtained using membranes alone, provided steps

were taken to ensure room for the regenerating tissues (Tinti and Vincenzi 1990). On the other hand, current research on growth factors (Williams 1990) has provided evidence that these biologic mediators obtain the same amount of periodontal regeneration with or without membranes. This finding would support the hypothesis that the biologic effect could contribute, at least partly, to the regeneration on recessions treated by FFSS plus membranes. To determine this, experimental treatment with membranes, associated or not with FFSS, would be needed. In such an experiment the mechanical problem should be solved by strictly mechanical devices.

## Future directions

There are several promising areas of research for the use of biologic mediators in guided tissue regeneration procedures: coronally positioned flaps for furcations, ridge augmentation, horizontal resorption, and implant surgery.

### Coronally positioned flaps

Encouraging clinical results have been obtained by treating class II furcation involvements in mandibular molars by a regenerative surgical technique consisting of coronally positioned flaps (Gantes et al 1988; Martin et al 1988). Because the few cases of class III furcations that we had the opportunity to treat by GTR plus FFSS were successful, one could expect that a combination of coronally positioned flap and FFSS would yield interesting outcomes. This association has already been tried on four cases of class II furcation involvement with satisfactory results (Fig 12-12). Experimental trials on class III furcations are needed before clinical application can be considered.

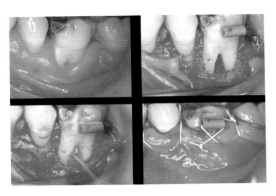

Fig 12-12 Treatment of a class II furcation involvement by means of coronally positioned flap and fibrin-fibronectin sealing system without membranes.

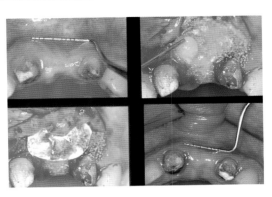

Fig 12-13 Ridge augmentation: the hydroxyapatite mixed with fibrin-fibronectin sealing system maintains the space for regeneration and supports the membrane. *Bottom right:* Healing after 8 weeks.

## Ridge augmentation

Experimental application of GTR by Seibert and Nyman (1990) to reconstruct localized ridge defects in dogs resulted in bone formation to fill the defect after 90 days. In ridge augmentation procedures, the FFSS could provide additional support and stability for the membrane during the early phase of would healing while maintaining room for the regenerating bone. Nine patients with localized buccal ridge deformities were treated using a combination of membranes, resorbable filling material (calcium carbonate), and FFSS (Cortellini et al 1993b) (Fig 12-13). One year after the treatment, the horizontal component of the ridge deformities was almost completely corrected in all the patients. However, consistent and predictable results were not obtained in correcting the vertical component of the defects, which were only partially filled in the vertical direction. Experimental and clinical research is needed to assess the possibility and the amount of improvement the use of biologic mediators can generate.

## Horizontal bone resorption

The treatment of horizontal bone resorption by GTR procedures has thus far been deceiving. However, ridge augmentation has been obtained in edentulous areas (Seibert and Nyman 1990), and different periodontal defects can be treated successfully by GTR procedures. Therefore, there should be no biologic reason that horizontal bone resorption is refractory to GTR. Rather, the obstacle should be a technical one. The FFSS could be useful in overcoming the mechanical problems, and biologic mediators could enhance the predictability of such treatments, by inducing or enhancing the coronal migration of periodontal ligament cells, for example.

## Implant surgery

Guided tissue regeneration procedures are being tested in implant surgery to enlarge the crestal width, to lift the height of the crest, or to cope with the empty space in extraction sites (Dahlin et al 1989; Lazzara 1989; Nyman et al 1990). Melcher

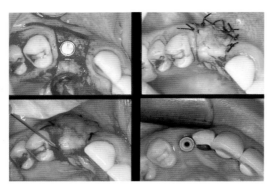

Fig 12-14 Endosseous implant (IMZ, Interpore International, Irvine, Calif) placement after traumatic loss of the maxillary right canine and lateral incisor in a 32-year-old woman. Fibrin-fibronectin sealing system is used to seal the wound, to minimize the risk of early infection. *Bottom right:* Healing after 6 months. The implant has now been working uneventfully for the past 3 years.

(1988) has already stressed the advantage of making the various implant surfaces most suitable for the tissues in front of them to obtain a stable interface as soon as possible. Sorption of fibronectin and other biologic mediators on the implant surface could be advantageous in the obtainment of a connective tissue interface prior to epithelial migration in critical applications. These include immediate posttraumatic or postextraction cases and cases of failure of a previous implant in the same site.

Because infection can cause implant failures, an additional advantage could be obtained using a FFSS, which provides a tight continuous seal of the wound along the entire incision line (Fig 12-14). This effect has already been exploited in neurosurgery to avoid postoperative infections when the transoral approach to the craniovertebral junction is used (Corona et al 1984). In the reported cases there were no fatalities. If the use of FFSS to create a seal against infection lowered the mortality

rate of this operation, the same procedure can also be expected to lower the failure rate of implants in the most critical applications, by preventing infection through the surgical incision.

## Conclusions

The biologic mediators contained in the fibrin-fibronectin sealing system have been used in regenerative procedures. Surgery was facilitated and shortened. The healing and maturation of the tissues were improved. In guided tissue regeneration procedures, the use of FFSS was associated with a satisfactory outcome even in the most critical cases. It is our opinion that the FFSS improves clinical results in many instances. However, it has still to be determined whether the clinical successes can be ascribed to the biologic mediators or to the mechanical features of the artificial clot. Because the cumulative effect is most satisfying, further research should be carried out in this field.

## References

Bartolucci EG, Pini Prato G. Preliminary observations on the use of a biologic sealing system (Tissucol®) in periodontal surgery. *J Periodontol* 1982;53:731–735.

Becker W, Becker BE, Prichard JP, Caffesse R, Rosenberg E, Giangrasso J. Root isolation for new attachment procedures: surgical and suturing method. Three case reports. *J Periodontol* 1987;58:819–826.

Caffesse RG, Holden MJ, Kon S, Nasjleti CE. The effect of citric acid and fibronectin application on healing following surgical treatment of naturally occurring periodontal disease in beagle dog. *J Clin Periodontol* 1985;12:578–590.

Caffesse RG, Kerry GJ, Chaves ES, et al. Clinical evaluation of the use of citric acid and autologous fibronectin in periodontal surgery. *J Periodontol* 1988;59:565–569.

Caffesse RG, Dominguez LE, Nasjleti C, Castelli WA, Morrison EC, Smith BA. Furcation defects in dog treated by guided tissue regeneration (GTR). *J Periodontol* 1990;61:45–50.

Caffesse R, Nasjleti C, Anderson G, Lopatin D, Smith B, Morrison E. Periodontal healing following guided tissue regeneration with citric acid and fibronectin application. *J Periodontol* 1991;62:21–29.

Caton JG, Polson AM, Pini Prato G, Bartolucci EG, Clauser C. Healing after application of tissue-adhesive material to denuded and citric acid-treated root surfaces. *J Periodontol* 1986;57: 385–390.

Corona C, Arena O, Fiumara E. *Atti del Convegno multidisciplinare sul Tissucol*. Pisa, Italy: Edizioni medicoscientifiche Immuno SpA; 1984:21–24.

Cortellini P, Pini Prato GP, Baldi C, Clauser C. Guided tissue regeneration with different materials. *Int J Periodont Rest Dent* 1990;10: 137–151.

Cortellini P, De Sanctis M, Pini Prato GP, Baldi C, Clauser C. Guided tissue regeneration procedure using a fibrin-fibronectin system in surgically induced recessions, in dogs. *Int J Periodont Rest Dent* 1991;11:151–153.

Cortellini P, Tonetti M, Pini Prato GP. Guided tissue regeneration in infrabony defects with and without a fibrin-fibronectin system: one year reentry procedure and X-ray evaluation (abstract). *J Periodontol* 1991;62:800.

Cortellini P, Pini Prato GP, Tonetti M. Periodontal regeneration of human infrabony defects. I. Clinical measures. *J Periodontol* 1993a;64:254–260.

Cortellini P, Pini Prato GP, Tonetti M. Periodontal regeneration of human infrabony defects. II. Reentry procedures and bone measures. *J Periodontol* 1993b;64:261–268.

Cortellini P, Bartolucci E, Clauser C, Pini Prato GP. Localized ridge augmentation using guided tissue regeneration in humans. A nine-case report. *J Clin Oral Impl Res* 1993c (In press).

Dahlin C, Sennerby L, Lekholm U, Linde A, Nyman S. Generation of new bone around titanium implants using a membrane technique: an experimental study in rabbits. *Int J Oral Maxillofac Implants* 1989;4:19–25.

Egelberg J. Regeneration and repair of periodontal tissues. *J Periodont Res* 1987;22:233–242.

Fernyhough W, Page RC. Attachment, growth, and synthesis by human gingival fibroblasts on demineralized or fibronectin–treated normal and diseased root surfaces. *J Periodontol* 1983;54: 133–140.

Gantes B, Martin M, Garrett S, Egelberg J. Treatment of periodontal furcation defects. Bone regeneration in mandibular class II defects. *J Clin Periodontol* 1988;15:232–239.

Gottlow J, Nyman S, Lindhe J, Karring T, Wennström J. New attachment formation in the human periodontium by guided tissue regeneration. Case reports. *J Clin Periodontol* 1986;13:604–616.

Lazzara RJ. Immediate implant placement into extraction sites: surgical and restorative advantages. *Int J Periodont Rest Dent* 1989;9:333–343.

Lynch SE, Nixon JC, Colvin RB, Antoniades HN. Role of platelet-derived growth factor in wound healing: synergistic effects with other growth factors. *Proc Nat Acad Sci USA* 1987;84:7696–7700.

Lynch SE, Williams RC, Polson AM, et al. A combination of platelet-derived and insulin-like growth factors enhances periodontal regeneration. *J Clin Periodont* 1989;16:545–548.

Martin, M, Gantes B, Garrett S, Egelberg J. Treatment of periodontal furcation defects. Review of the literature and description of a regenerative surgical technique. *J Clin Periodontol* 1988; 15:227–231.

Matras H, Kuderna H. Glueing nerve anastomoses with clotting substances. Transactions of the 6th *International Congress of Plastic and Reconstructive Surgery* 1975:134–138.

Melcher A. Summary of biological considerations. *J Dent Educ* 1988;52:812–814.

Mendieta C, Caravana C, Fine DH. Sorption of fibronectin to human root surface in vitro. *J Periodont* 1990;61:254–260.

Nasjleti CE, Caffesse RG, Castelli WA, Lopatin DE, Kowalski CJ. Effects of lyophilized autologous plasma on periodontal healing of replanted teeth. *J Periodontol* 1986;57:568–578.

Nyman S, Lindhe J, Karring T, Rylander H. New attachment following surgical treatment of human periodontal disease. *J Clin Periodontol* 1982; 9:290–296.

Nyman S, Lang PN, Buser D, Brägger U. Bone regeneration adjacent to titanium dental implants using guided tissue regeneration: a report of two cases. *Int J Oral Maxillofac Implants* 1990;5:9–14.

Pini Prato G, De Paoli S, Clauser C, Bartolucci E. On the use of a biologic sealing system (Tissucol®) in periodontal surgery. *Int J Periodont Rest Dent* 1983;3(4):49–60.

Pini Prato G, De Paoli S, Cortellini P, Zerosi C, Clauser C. On the use of a biologic sealing system (Tissucol®) in periodontal therapy. II. Histologic evaluation. *Int J Periodont Rest Dent* 1985;5(3):33–41.

Pini Prato GP, Clauser C, Cortellini P. The use of fibrin sealant (Tissucol/Tisseel) in periodontal surgery: clinical and histological evaluation. In: G Schlag, H Redl, eds. *Fibrin Sealant In Operative Medicine Plastic Surgery — Maxillofacial Surgery and Dental Surgery*. Berlin, Heidelberg, Germany: Springer Verlag; 1986;4:183–187.

Pini Prato GP, Cortellini P, Agudio G, Clauser C. Human fibrin glue versus sutures in periodontal surgery. *J Periodontol* 1987;58:426–431.

Pini Prato GP, Cortellini P, Clauser C. Fibrin and fibronectin sealing system in a guided tissue regeneration procedure. A case report. *J Periodontol* 1988;59:679–683.

Polson AM, Proye MP. Fibrin linkage: a precursor of new attachment. J Periodontol 1983;54: 141–147.

Pontoriero R, Nyman S, Lindhe J, Rosenberg E, Sanavi F. Guided tissue regeneration in the treatment of furcation defects in man. *J Clin Periodontol* 1987;14:618–620.

Pontoriero R, Lindhe J, Nyman S, Karring T, Rosenberg E, Sanavi F. Guided tissue regeneration in degree II furcation-involved mandibular molars. A clinical study. *J Clin Periodontol* 1988;15:247–254.

Ripamonti U, Petit J-C, Lemmer J, Austin JC. Regeneration of the connective tissue attachment on surgically exposed roots using a fibrin-fibronectin adhesive system. An experimental study on the baboon *(Papio ursinus)*. *J Periodont Res* 1987;22:320–326.

Schlag G, Redl H. *Fibrin Sealant In Operative Medicine.* Berlin, Heidelberg, Germany: Springer Verlag; 1986.

Seelich T. Tissucol (Immuno, Vienna): biochemistry and methods of application. *J Head Neck Pathol* 1982;3:65–69.

Seibert J, Nyman S. Localized ridge augmentation in dogs: a pilot study using membranes and hydroxyapatite. *J Periodontol* 1990;61:157–165.

Smith B, Caffesse R, Nasjleti C, Kon S, Castelli W. Effects of citric acid and fibronectin and laminin application in treating periodontitis. *J Clin Periodontol* 1987;14:396–402.

Terranova VP, Hic S, Franzetti L, Lyall RM, Wikesjö UME. A biochemical approach to periodontal regeneration. AFSCM: assays for specific cell migration. *J Periodontol* 1987;58:247–257.

Terranova VP, Martin GR. Molecular factors determing gingival tissue interaction with structures. *J Periodont Res* 1982;17:530–257.

Terranova VP, Odziemiec C, Tweden KS, Spadone DP. Repopulation of dentin surfaces by periodontal ligament cells and endothelial cells. *J Periodontol* 1989;60:293–301.

Terranova VP, Wikesjö UME. Extracellular matrices and polypeptide growth factors as mediators of functions of cells of the periodontium. A review. *J Periodontol* 1987;58:371–380.

Tinti C, Vincenzi G. Il trattamento delle recessioni gengivali con la tecnica di "rigenerazione guidata dei tessuti" mediante membrane Gore-Tex(R). Variante clinica. *Quintessence Int* (Italian) 1990; 6:465–468.

Williams RC. Current problems in periodontology. Presented at the 5th International Congress of the Italian Society for Periodontology; February 15–17, 1990; Rome, Italy.

Wikesjö UME, Claffey N, Christersson LA, et al. Repair of periodontal furcation defects in beagle dogs following reconstructive surgery including root surface demineralization with tetracycline hydrochloride and topical fibronectin application. *J Clin Periodontol* 1988;15:73–80.

Yeung S, Boyatzis S. The use of autologous fibronectin in the surgical repair of through-and-through furcation lesions in man. A pilot study. *J Clin Periodontol* 1990;17:321–323.

# Index